100 ORGANIC SKIN CARE RECIPES

100 ORGANIC SKIN CARE RECIPES

Make Your Own Fresh and
Fabulous Organic Beauty Products

JESSICA RESS

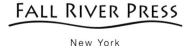

FALL RIVER PRESS

New York

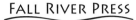

FALL RIVER PRESS

New York

An Imprint of Sterling Publishing Co., Inc.
1166 Avenue of the Americas
New York, NY 10036

Fall River Press and the distinctive Fall River Press logo are registered trademarks of
Barnes & Noble, Inc.

ISBN 978-1-4351-6403-1

For information about custom editions, special sales, and premium and corporate purchases,
please contact Sterling Special Sales at 800-805-5489 or specialsales@sterlingpublishing.com.

Manufactured in China

2 4 6 8 10 9 7 5 3

www.sterlingpublishing.com

Photography by Jessica Ress and Diane Harrison. Images on pages 21, 24, 35, 36, 51, 57, 60, 78, 82,
85, 93, 94, 99, 101, 106, 122, 135, 138, 147, 158, 163, 168, 177, 182, 188, 193 by Adams Media.

CONTENTS

Introduction 9

CHAPTER 1

**WHAT YOU NEED TO KNOW
ABOUT SKIN CARE** 11

CHAPTER 2

FACIAL CARE 15

Acai Berry Facial Scrub 16

Shea Butter Lip Balm 17

Maca Vitality Scrub 18

Ayurvedic Facial Cleansing Grains 19

Gentle Glow Washing Grains 20

Clarifying Toner 22

Oil Cleanser for Clogged Pores 23

Rooibos Rose Toner 26

Balancing Facial Moisturizer 28

Vital Facial Moisturizer 29

Luxurious Vita-E Facial Oil 31

Green Tea Eye Cream 32

Spa Facial Steam for Normal to Oily Skin . . 33

Soothing Herbal Steam 34

Chocolate Lip Scrub 37

Green Tea and Adzuki Cleansing Grains . . . 38

CHAPTER 3

FACIAL MASKS 41

Yerba Flax Face-Food Mask 42

Radiant Orange Mask 43

Green Clay Rose Milk Mask 44

Clarifying Probiotic Moisture Surge 46

Carrot-Coconut NutraMoist Mask 47

Aztec Honey and Wine Mask 49

Coco-Superfruit Mask 50

Chia Coconut Superfood Mask 52

Soothing Oil-Free Mask 53

Manuka and Parsley Lightening
Acne Mask 55

Go Green Moisture Mask 56

Agave Rose Anti-Aging Mask 58

Rainforest Elixir Mask 59

Fresh Petals Mask 61

CHAPTER 4

BODY SCRUBS AND WASHES 63

Olive Butter Scrub 64

Javanese Gold Body Scrub 65

Sugar Chai Honey Scrub 66

Herb Garden Body Scrub 69

Gentle Oatmeal Wash 70

Mocha Latte Scrub 71

Citrus Blast Body Scrub 72

Vanilla, Bourbon, and Honey Scrub 75

Almond Moisture Scrub 76

Valencia Coffee Scrub 79

Floral Oatmeal Wash 80

Lemon Poppy Seed Scrub 83

Invigorating Ginger Citrus Body Wash 84

Shea Butter Body Wash 86

Honey Coconut Body Wash 87

CHAPTER 5

BODY BUTTERS AND OILS 89

Body Butter Bars 90

Healing Comfrey Salve 92

Gardener's Herbal Balm 95

Whipped Shea Body Butter 96

Lovely Body Butter 97

Coco-Spice Body Butter 100

Luxurious Body Oil 102

Sore Muscle Massage Oil 103

Warm Cinnamon Massage Oil 104

Cuticle Saver Treatment 107

CHAPTER 6

BATHS 109

Coconut, Lime, and Rose Petals Bath 110

Mermaid Bath 111

Sunshine C Bath 112

Bath Melts 114

Moisturizing Bath Salts 116

Bath Fizzies 117

Angel Soak for Cold and Flu 120

Ideal Luxury Bath 123

Chamomile and Oat Super
Soothe-Me Bath 125

CHAPTER 7

INFUSIONS 129

Green Tea–Infused Oil 130

Chai Spice–Infused Oil 132

Rosemary-Infused Oil 133

Vanilla-Infused Oil 136

Fresh Comfrey Oil 137

Fresh Herbal Oil 139

Lavender-Infused Oil. 140

Sweet Dreamtime–Infused Oil 142

Layered Lavender Flower Water 143

Old-Fashioned Rosewater 145

Aromatic Vanilla Infusion 146

CHAPTER 8

WHOLE-BODY SPA TREATMENTS. . . 149

Head-to-Toe Pumpkin Mask 150

Glowing Goddess Face and Body Mask. . . 152

Coconut Rice Conditioning Exfoliant. 154

Ambrosia Face and Body Mask 155

Vanilla Isle Perfume 156

Blushing Bride Ubtan Exfoliant 157

Detoxifying Seaweed Body Wrap 160

Fizzy Mojito Foot Spa 162

Soothing Scalp and Hair Treatment 164

Jasmine Hair Finishing Oil. 166

Sunrise Spa Water. 167

Cucumber De-Puffer Spa Water 169

Strawberry Super C Sipper 170

Quick Coconut Cantaloupe Cooler 172

Rosy Green Tea Spa Water 173

CHAPTER 9

SUN CARE 175

Sun-Kissed Pre-Tanning Body Scrub 176

Yogurt Lavender Comfort Body Mask
and Bath. 179

Avo-Oat After-Sun Face and Body Mask. . . 180

Calming Antioxidant Skin Quencher 181

Cooling Anti-Itch Paste 183

Soothe-My-Sunburn Bath. 184

Healing Sunburn Spray and Compress . . . 186

Cucumber Rose Sunburn Relief. 189

Sun Protection Lotion Stick. 190

Beachy Babe Hair Spray 192

Appendix A: Essential Oil Blends 195

Appendix B: Bonus Facial Treatments . . . 197

Appendix C: Glossary of Ingredients 203

Metric Conversion Chart. 214

Index 216

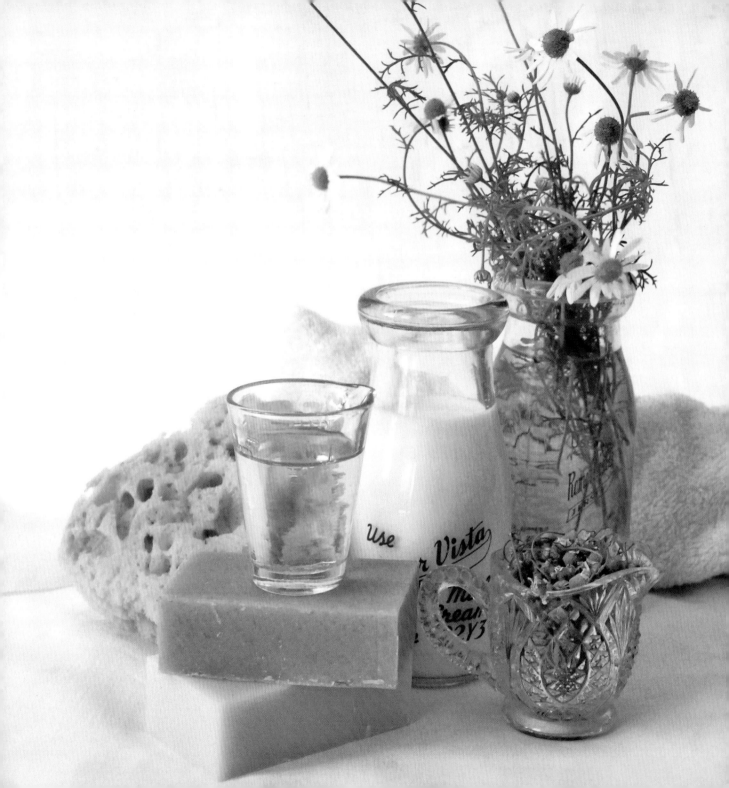

INTRODUCTION

Do you want to slather your lips with an edible Chocolate Lip Scrub? Lay in the bathtub and drift away on the clean scent of an Invigorating Ginger Citrus Body Wash? Wrap yourself in the luxury of a Glowing Goddess Face and Body Mask?

Throughout *100 Organic Skin Care Recipes*, you'll find amazing skin care products that will take your skin—and your mind, body, and spirit—to places they've never been before. Filled with all-natural ingredients like fresh herbs, flowers, honey, shea butter, or a unique essential oil blend (Appendix A), each recipe gives you the opportunity to mix up your own personalized batch of skin care that is free of the hazardous chemicals found in store-bought brands. Each ingredient has been chosen for its health and beauty benefits, detailed in the Glossary of Ingredients (Appendix C). Each recipe contains step-by-step instructions that teach you how to use oils, herbs, and other organic ingredients to create nourishing products for healthy skin. In Appendix B you will find facial care treatment plans to help you create a natural beauty routine that's perfect for your unique skin type.

These recipes—from the Layered Lavender Flower Water to the Lemon Poppy Seed Scrub—are inspired by the simple things in life that make you feel alive. The gorgeous flowers blooming in the garden. The fresh and tangy scent of fresh fruit. A softly scented breeze. Nature provides an amazing world full of divinely decadent and infinitely therapeutic ingredients for you to create these exquisite spa products. Each recipe is organic, natural, and chemical-free. Because why would you put something on your body that you wouldn't put in it?

Each one of these replenishing products is special and unique, and they are deceptively easy to create—which means they make impressive gifts for holidays, birthdays, or any other special occasion. You can make these skin care recipes in your own kitchen with the tools and ingredients you have on hand. Most of the ingredients can be found at the natural food store or farmer's market. There are a few specialty ingredients or types of packaging that are easily found online with a quick Internet search.

I formulate these gorgeous recipes with love. It's simply what I do. I hope that shows. And I hope you will love discovering these creations as much as I enjoyed putting them together for you. I created space for you to add your personal touches with decorative packaging, layering scents, and dreaming up fabulous ways to plan an absolutely divine Home Spa Day. I humbly suggest that you make these recipes with focused healing intention and lots of love. Those two little things are my secret and favorite ingredients and I include them in all of my recipes.

May your skin glow like the petals of a flower and smell as sweet . . .

xoxo
SpaGoddess

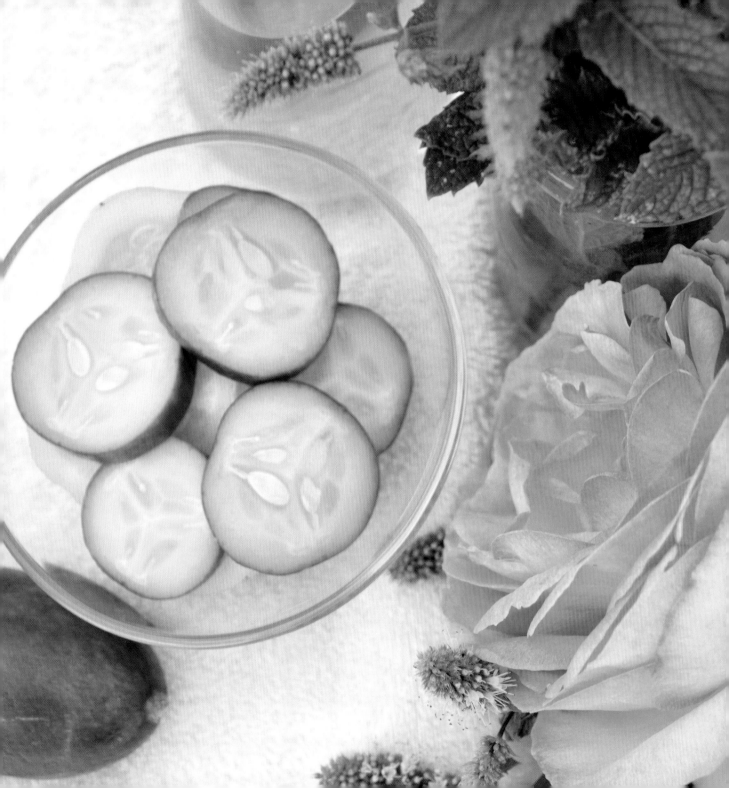

CHAPTER 1

WHAT YOU NEED TO KNOW ABOUT SKIN CARE

Have you ever not washed your face before bed and awakened to a bunch of little pimples? Probably. Have you ever eaten a bunch of French fries, chocolate, or junk food and had your skin erupt in an epic breakout in the next day or two? Who hasn't! The relationship between your skin and your body is symbiotic, mutually reliant, and interdependent. It's important to realize that the foundation for healthy, radiant skin starts on the inside.

Your skin is the largest and fastest-growing organ of your body and accounts for 6 to 10 percent of your body weight. All of your cells require good nutrition, proper hydration, oxygenation, and detoxification to thrive. What you put on your skin is just as important as what you put in your body. With this in mind, healthy skin can be achieved by making positive, well-considered choices in relation to your mind, body, and spirit. In addition to your skin care regimen, you want to pay attention to additional factors that can contribute to healthy skin, including:

♦ *Sun exposure*

♦ *Eating habits*

♦ *Hydration*

♦ *Exercise*

♦ *Environmental pollutants*

All of these factors combine with your genetic makeup and overall wellness to comprise the health of your skin. And while skin care products can help combat and correct some of the inherent issues and skin conditions, it is best to think of healthy skin holistically, as part of a completely healthy you. After all, a healthy you is a happy you. Keeping that in mind, let's take a look at the simple things that make the recipes in this book decadent, healthy, and inspiring!

Fresh Ingredients

Throughout the book, you will find many recipes that call for fresh fruits, vegetables, herbs, and flowers. Just like the food you eat, these natural skin care ingredients are best used when fresh. Fresh ingredients are at their peak of vitality, and plants that are picked at their peak and used immediately will contribute their nutrient-rich vitality to the recipe. You'll also find superfoods in quite a few of the skin care recipes due to their high concentrations of vital phytonutrients that greatly benefit your skin. But no matter which recipe you make, remember that fresh is best!

Make the Right Size

You'll find both single use and large batch recipes throughout the book. Most of the single use recipes are made with fresh, perishable skin food ingredients and are intended to be used immediately. The larger batch recipes can be made ahead of time and used in your daily facial care routines and weekly home spa rituals. You'll also find a variety of recipes that make multiples, such as the Bath Fizzies and Body Butter Bars that you can creatively package as party favors and gorgeous handmade gifts for your loved ones.

Natural and Organic

For me, organic is a lifestyle. My skin care company, Angel Face Botanicals, was founded on organic principles. My main goal when I started my skin care company was to offer consumers highly effective, ultra-luxurious botanically based products with incredible natural scents. The recipes you'll find throughout this book allow you to create your own natural and deliciously scented products in your own home. So, when shopping for the ingredients, keep the quality of the final product in mind. Your creation will only be "organic" if the raw materials you source are organic. Unfortunately, if the ingredient isn't organic, then you can almost guarantee that it was grown with synthetic fertilizers and pesticides

and/or is a genetically modified ingredient. I make conscious choices to limit my exposure to manmade chemicals in our environment, and I encourage you to do the same. I am a firm believer in the benefits of organic farming for our food and water supply, for our skin care products, and for the overall health and well-being of our planet Earth and all of her inhabitants.

Aromatherapy and Herbal Skin Care

Many of the skin care recipes in the book will benefit all skin types, and others are intended for specific skin types and conditions. You many wonder how the same facial cleanser could benefit dry, maturing skin and also be good for oily, acne-prone skin. Well, many botanical ingredients are adaptogens, or balancers. This means that, as the plant substance makes its way through the bloodstream, it attends to the specific needs of the individual person. For example, a product can be either calming or stimulating depending on the person who uses it. While this concept is not widely accepted in Western medical philosophy, it has been effectively employed for thousands of years in traditional Chinese medicine, as well as Ayurvedic medicine, which has a similar concept called *rasayana*. Additionally, all skin types benefit from increased cellular health and regeneration. Many of the skin care preparations included in this book are formulated as tonic skin conditioners to promote vitality and support balanced oil production in all skin types.

The Home Spa

It is important to set aside some "me time" every once in a while to enjoy a home spa ritual. This is a completely self-directed nurturing experience that benefits every aspect of you, including physical and mental detoxification, stress reduction, raising self-esteem, and increased overall health and well-being. You may also want to have friends over for a home spa party where you cook up a fabulous array of homemade skin care treats to enjoy as a group.

Whether you create a meditative solitary spa day or a boisterous home spa party with friends, the goal is to pamper yourself, nurture your skin, revive your spirit, and restore balance to your entire being. During these home spa sessions, deliberately leave your daily worries at the door and surrender to relaxation and replenishment. This is your "me time" to nurture health and vitality in your mind, body, and spirit. You have committed to a sensory journey with the sole purpose of making positive improvements to your overall well-being. Create the home spa recipes in this book for your enjoyment, your beautification, your stress release, your joy.

Above All, Love Yourself

True beauty comes from being happy and feeling beautiful. Using fabulous skin care and home spa products just feels good, makes your skin happy, and makes your heart glow too. With that in mind, here is my favorite and most valuable beauty secret, the simple thing that you can do every day to enhance your inner glow and outer radiance. Are you ready for this? All you have to do is look in the mirror at least once each day and say to yourself: "You are so beautiful. I love you!" If this seems hard, do it anyway! The more you do this, the easier it will become. Just take a deep breath, inhale love, and exhale peace. This simple process actually goes really deep, to the core of your being. It can bring emotions and deeper issues to the surface. And that is

a good thing! Your heartfelt emotions are a beautiful reflection of you.

"You are so beautiful. I love you!" Just simply say those words to yourself, every day. Soon after you start this, people in your life will notice a new sparkle in your eye or a bounce in your step. Don't be surprised if you start to receive random compliments on the peace and radiance that you carry. And it comes from making this simple statement your reality. The more you say this, the more you feel it; believe it, and live this truth deep down in your core: You are so beautiful!

The point of the skin care recipes and the advice you'll find throughout the book is to help you feel beautiful. Because when you feel beautiful, you project a beautiful, happy vibration out into the world. The simple and enjoyable act of preparing these recipes is nurturing in and of itself. Making these recipes nurtures your creative side and reinforces a healthful lifestyle that you can feel good about. The "me time" that you proactively set aside for a home spa experience is a loving, nurturing gesture of self-love. And you, my beautiful darling, deserve every minute of it!

So without further ado, let's take a look at the recipes that will enrich your body, your mind, and your spirit . . .

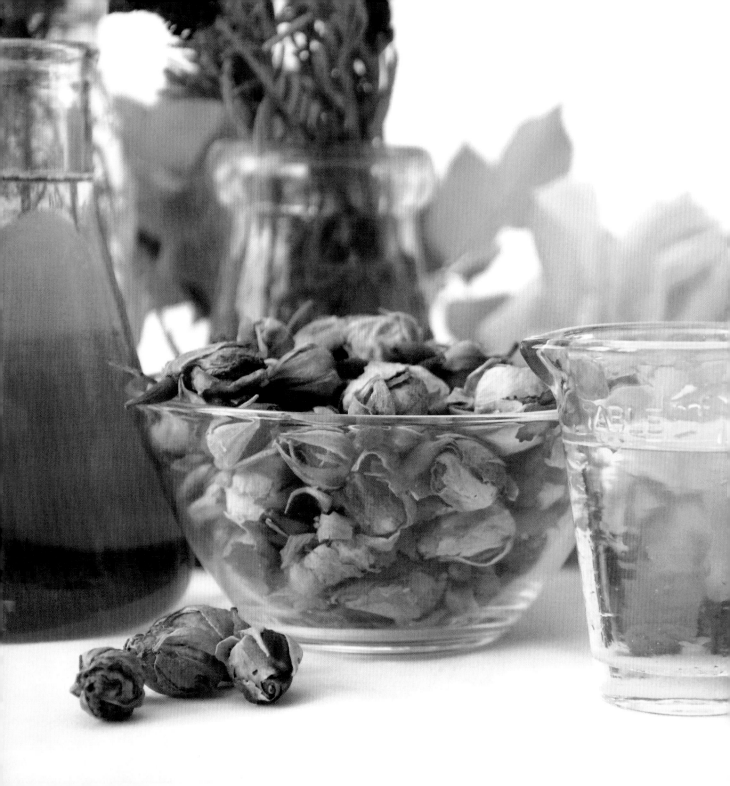

CHAPTER 2

FACIAL CARE

Taking good care of your facial skin is quite simple when you break it down to the basics—cleanse, tone, and moisturize your face twice per day, every day. The first step is a cleanser such as the Ayurvedic Facial Cleansing Grains to gently clean the dirt, sweat, oil, and environmental buildup from the surface of your skin to prevent redness, irritation, clogged pores, and dull, ashy skin. Next, you'll use a facial toner like the Rooibos Rose Toner or the Clarifying Toner found in this chapter to correct the pH level on the surface of your skin and close and minimize your pores so they don't fill up with gunk. The final crucial step is to use a facial moisturizer like the Balancing Facial Moisturizer that will leave your skin with a nourishing moisture layer that addresses the needs of your specific skin type. Why use a moisturizer? Well, without one, your skin will go haywire trying to overcorrect, causing overly dry or overly oily skin, which exacerbates redness, breakouts, and clogged pores.

Throughout this chapter you'll find everything you need to follow these three basic steps—plus some luxury skin treatment products such as the Chocolate Lip Scrub, Soothing Herbal Steam, and Green Tea Eye Cream. So say goodbye to red, irritated, broken-out, dry, or oily skin and say hello to healthy, clean, clear, and radiant skin.

Acai Berry FACIAL SCRUB

Acai berries have a remarkable concentration of trace minerals, amino acids, essential fatty acids, phytosterols, and antioxidants that help the skin regenerate, speeding up the healing process for acneic skin. The cornmeal and kaolin in this recipe act like a sponge that absorbs excess oil while drawing out toxins and impurities from your pores. The oat flour adds a soothing, moisturizing component. This recipe is highly beneficial to all skin types, especially oily and acne prone.

YIELDS: *1 quart*

½ cup acai berry powder

½ cup oat flour

½ cup finely ground cornmeal

½ cup kaolin clay

What you will need: face mask, quart-size canning jar with lid, spice jar with sifter cap (optional)

1 To Make: Before you begin, find a protective face mask, or tie a bandana to cover your nose and mouth, to avoid breathing the powdered ingredients. Carefully place all of the ingredients into the canning jar. Close the lid tightly and shake well to blend to a uniform powder. Let stand for 5 minutes or so, letting the dust settle into the jar.

2 To Store: Store this dry facial scrub in a spice jar with a sifter cap. To fill the jar, make a funnel by rolling up a piece of paper. Twist one end to open wide enough to fit into the spice jar, and the other wider to funnel in the powder. Tape it together and spoon the powder into the jar a little at a time. Once the jar is full, replace the sifter and cap, and this scrub is ready to use! You can also store this scrub in the quart jar or transfer to a smaller jar, using a clean dry spoon to dispense the facial scrub for each use. Keep the lid tightly closed and store for up to a year.

3 To Use: To use, simply tap out a bit of the powder into the palm of your hand and mix with water added a tiny bit at a time until a paste forms. Then softly cleanse your face using small circular motions. Rinse with warm water and follow with toner and moisturizer.

Shea Butter
LIP BALM

This positively luscious lip balm provides relief and a healing boost for dry, chapped lips. Shea butter, sweet almond oil, coconut oil, and beeswax form a perfect nurturing barrier to protect your lips against chapping, helping them stay super soft and super kissable. Find some cute containers and this recipe makes a fun gift too. To add some color, melt a pea-size amount—or more!—of your favorite lipstick in this balm. Enjoy!

YIELDS: *1 ounce*

1 teaspoon grated beeswax

2 teaspoons shea butter

1 teaspoon coconut oil

2 teaspoons sweet almond oil

Pinch of stevia, optional

10 drops of essential oils, optional

What you will need: measuring spoons, double boiler, tiny whisk, rubber spatula, lip balm tubes, jars or tins to hold a 1-ounce batch of lip balm

1 **To Make:** Start the double boiler on medium heat. Once it reaches a boil, reduce heat to simmer. Place the beeswax and shea butter in the top of the double boiler and cover. Simmer until melted, stirring occasionally. Add the coconut oil and stir until melted. To preserve the beneficial nutrients, do not overheat. Remove from heat, take the top pan off the double boiler, and dry with a towel so no water drips into your melted butter. Add the sweet almond oil and stevia, if desired, and stir with the whisk. Next, stir in the essential oils, scraping any of the hardened cooled mixture off the sides of the pot and back into the melted oils. Pour into your jars, cover with plastic wrap, and let stand undisturbed for 4 hours or overnight. Put the lids on tightly and label with contents and date. Note: If the mixture hardens too much before you can pour it, gently melt it again in the double boiler.

2 **To Store:** Store in a cool dry place away from direct sunlight. Use within a year.

3 **To Use:** To use, remove a small amount from the jar with your fingertip and spread onto your lips.

Maca
VITALITY SCRUB

Give your skin a good dose of vitamins and antioxidants with this exfoliating blend of maca and cacao. Topically applied, these South American superfoods are high in regenerative essential fatty acids, proteins, vitamins, and minerals, which help improve the tone and texture of your skin. Use 1–2 times per week when your skin needs a vitamin-boosted exfoliation.

YIELDS: *about 1 pint*

½ cup maca powder

¼ cup coconut flour

½ cup kaolin clay

½ cup fine granulated sugar

1 tablespoon raw cocoa/cacao powder

What you will need: face mask, pint-size canning jar with lid, spice jar with sifter cap (optional)

1 **To Make:** Before you begin, find a protective face mask, or tie a bandana to cover your nose and mouth, to avoid breathing the powders. Carefully place all of the powdered ingredients into the canning jar. Close the lid tightly and shake well to blend to a uniform powder. Let stand for 5 minutes or so, letting the dust settle into the jar.

2 **To Store:** Store this dry facial scrub in a spice jar with a sifter cap. To fill the jar, make a funnel by rolling up a piece of paper. Twist one end to open wide enough to fit into the spice jar, and the other wider to funnel in the powder. Tape it together and spoon the powder into the jar a little at a time. Once the jar is full, replace the sifter and cap, and this scrub is ready to use! You can also store these in the pint jar or transfer to a smaller jar, using a clean dry spoon to dispense the cleansing grains for each use. Keep the lid tightly closed and store for up to a year.

3 **To Use:** To use, simply tap out a bit of the powder into the palm of your hand and mix with water added a tiny bit at a time until a paste forms. Then softly cleanse your face using small circular motions. Rinse with warm water and follow with toner and moisturizer.

Ayurvedic
FACIAL CLEANSING GRAINS

Facial cleansing grains are part of a centuries-old beauty regimen popular in India, Japan, and other Asian cultures. This powdered facial cleanser combines natural ingredients to gently exfoliate and remove excess oil and dirt without stripping your skin's natural beneficial moisture. Just add water and your skin is left clean, smooth, radiant, and glowing.

YIELDS: *1 quart*

½ cup almond meal

½ cup rose petal powder

1 tablespoon turmeric

2 teaspoons orange peel powder

½ cup chickpea flour

½ cup kaolin clay

½ cup brown rice flour

½ teaspoon cinnamon

What you will need: face mask, quart-size canning jar with lid, spice jar with sifter cap (optional)

HELPFUL HINTS

Avoid getting undiluted turmeric onto your skin, as it may stain.

❶ To Make: Before you begin, find a protective face mask, or tie a bandana to cover your nose and mouth, to avoid breathing the powders. Carefully place all of the powdered ingredients into the canning jar. You may want to consider sifting the brown rice flour, as there are usually some larger rice grains remaining, which can be a little rough on the skin. Close the lid tightly and shake well to blend to a uniform powder. Let stand for 5 minutes or so, letting the dust settle into the jar.

❷ To Store: Store this dry facial scrub in a spice jar with a sifter cap. To fill the jar, make a funnel by rolling up a piece of paper. Twist one end to open wide enough to fit into the spice jar, and the other wider to funnel in the powder. Tape it together and spoon the powder into the jar a little at a time. Once the jar is full, replace the sifter and cap, and this scrub is ready to use! You can also store these in the quart jar or transfer to a smaller jar, using a clean dry spoon to dispense the cleansing grains for each use. Keep the lid tightly closed and store for up to a year.

❸ To Use: To use, simply tap out a bit of the powder into the palm of your hand and mix with water added a tiny bit at a time until a paste forms. Then softly cleanse your face using small circular motions. Rinse with warm water and follow with toner and moisturizer.

Gentle Glow
WASHING GRAINS

This simple blend of soothing, moisturizing ingredients cleanses and exfoliates even the most sensitive skin. Oats are widely regarded as an ideal ingredient for sensitive and easily irritated skin because oatmeal nourishes, moisturizes, and gently exfoliates the skin, absorbing excess oil and dirt.

YIELDS: *1¾ cups*

¼ **cup rose petal powder**

¾ **cup oat flour**

½ **cup kaolin clay**

¼ **cup powdered milk**

What you will need: face mask, pint-size canning jar with lid, spice jar with sifter cap (optional)

1 **To Make:** Before you begin, find a protective face mask, or tie a bandana to cover your nose and mouth, to avoid breathing the powders. Carefully place all of the powdered ingredients into the canning jar. You may want to consider sifting the oat flour, as there are usually some larger pieces of oats remaining, which can be a little rough on delicate facial skin. Close the lid tightly and shake well to blend to a uniform powder. Let stand for 5 minutes or so, letting the dust settle into the jar.

2 **To Store:** Store this dry facial scrub in a spice jar with a sifter cap. To fill the jar, make a funnel by rolling up a piece of paper. Twist one end to open wide enough to fit into the spice jar, and the other wider to funnel in the powder. Tape it together and spoon the powder into the jar a little at a time. Once the jar is full, replace the sifter and cap, and this scrub is ready to use! You can also store these in the pint jar or transfer to a smaller jar, using a clean dry spoon to dispense the cleansing grains for each use. Keep the lid tightly closed and store for up to a year.

3 **To Use:** To use, simply tap out a bit of the powder into the palm of your hand and mix with water added a tiny bit at a time until a paste forms. Then softly cleanse your face using small circular motions. Rinse with warm water and follow with toner and moisturizer.

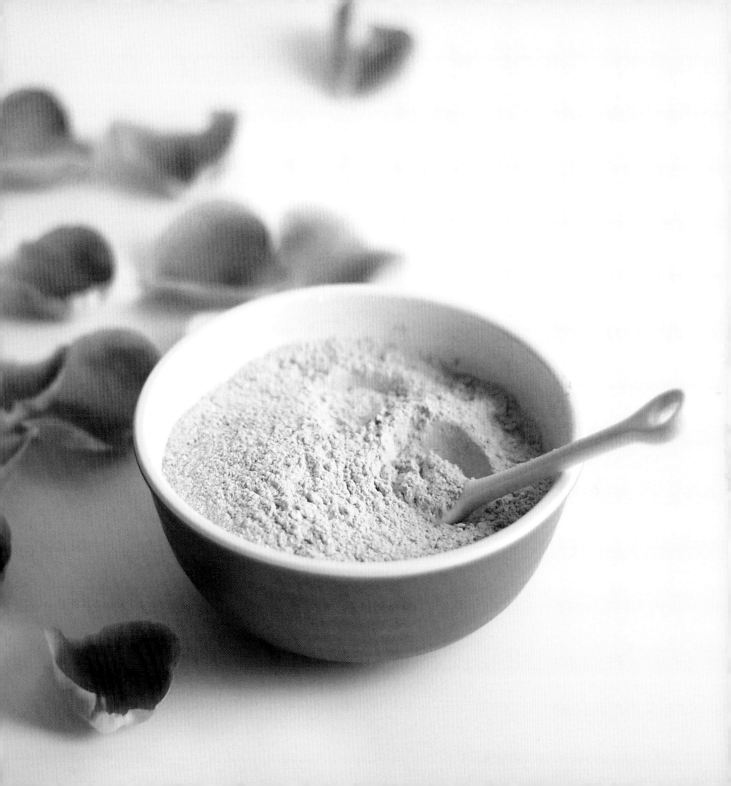

Clarifying TONER

Apple cider vinegar contains natural alpha-hydroxy acids, which work to slough off dead skin cells and lighten discolorations, including sun and age spots. This Clarifying Toner balances your skin's pH, removes built-up oil and grime, and closes and tightens pores, reducing their size. This formula is beneficial for normal to oily, combination, and acne-prone skin types.

YIELDS: *4 ounces*

2 tablespoons witch hazel

2 teaspoons raw apple cider vinegar

2 tablespoons distilled water

3 tablespoons Layered Lavender Flower Water (see Chapter 7) or lavender hydrosol (flower water)

What you will need: funnel, 4-ounce bottle and cap or mister top

1. **To Make:** Using the funnel, pour all of the ingredients into the bottle. Cap tightly and shake well.

2. **To Store:** Store in bottle and use within 1–2 months, or store in the refrigerator to extend the shelf life to 6 months.

3. **To Use:** Use twice per day after cleansing. Moisten a cotton pad and gently sweep over facial skin to remove the last traces of dirt, oil, and makeup. Follow with moisturizer and serum.

OIL CLEANSER
for Clogged Pores

This recipe is an advanced formulation for acne-prone skin that uses the basic principles of the *oil-cleansing method,* where the oil and dirt that are clogging your pores are drawn out, hardened plugs and all, and replaced with a healthy amount of beneficial botanical oils. You see, in the chemistry of skin care, oil dissolves oil. That may sound counterintuitive, but it's true. Use this cleanser once per week for clean, clear pores and progressively fewer blemishes.

YIELDS: *4 ounces*

4 tablespoons hazelnut oil

2 vitamin E capsules

6 drops tea tree essential oil

4 drops lavender essential oil

2 drops chamomile essential oil

1 tablespoon castor oil

1 tablespoon Rosemary-Infused Oil (see Chapter 7)

4 tablespoons grapeseed oil

What you will need: funnel, dark-colored 4-ounce bottle—one with a cap or pump top is ideal

❶ **To Make:** Place the funnel over your bottle and add the hazelnut oil. Pierce the vitamin E capsules and squeeze them out into the bottle, discarding the gel caps. Add the essential oils. Next, add the castor oil and Rosemary-Infused Oil, and fill up the bottle with grapeseed oil. Shake for a minute or so to blend.

❷ **To Store:** Store out of direct sunlight in bottle. Will keep for up to 6 months.

❸ **To Use:** Oil cleansers are best used at night, when your skin is in need of a deeper cleaning. Shake well before use, as the heavier oils may settle to the bottom. Start with dry rather than wet skin. Massage a pump or two into your skin using gentle circular, upward strokes. It is completely worth it to take the few extra minutes to massage areas of wrinkles and clogged pores for at least 3 minutes and up to 10 minutes. Avoid any active blemishes or recent eruptions. The longer you massage, the more debris you will feel (i.e., de-clogged pore gunk). It's gross, but fabulous, right?

(continued on page 25)

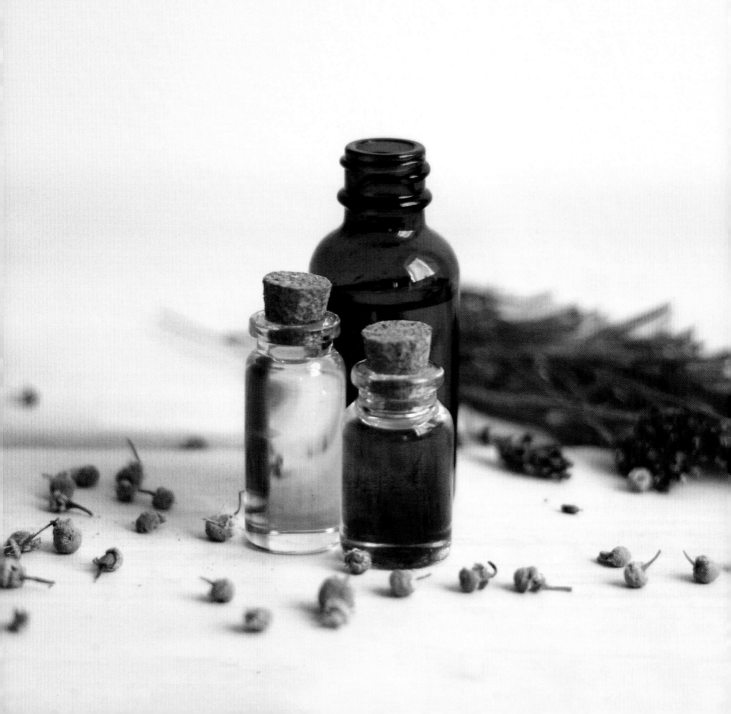

④ Next, run hot water over a washcloth. Wring the cloth out a bit, letting it cool so it's not too hot. Set the cloth on your face, steaming the oil, dirt, makeup, and grime out of your pores, then gently wipe the oil, dirt, and grime off your face. Rinse out the cloth well and repeat the steaming process 2–5 times. Use a few times per week, up to once per day as a facial cleanser. Start with once per week, working your way up in frequency depending on how your skin responds.

HELPFUL HINTS

Some people can use oil cleansers daily, but it's a once a week treatment for others. The oil cleanser draws the deeper toxins out to the surface, so do not be surprised if a few pimples form. These are not newly created, but were pre-existing, laying low, waiting to be brought to the surface to heal. This cleans out the deeper dermal layers of your skin, which is a necessary step for sustained clear, pimple-free skin. Be aware that you should not use an oil cleanser too often or it will dry out your skin.

Rooibos
ROSE TONER

Aloe Vera and Rosewater are soothing, hydrating, and conditioning. Rooibos is a powerful antioxidant that is high in vitamins and minerals including zinc and vitamin D. It also contains superoxide dismutase (SOD), an enzyme and amazingly effective antioxidant that attacks free radicals. This Rooibos Rose Toner balances your skin's pH, removes built-up oil and grime, and closes and tightens pores, reducing size and appearance. This formula is beneficial for normal to dry, combination, acne-prone, rosacea-prone, and maturing skin types.

YIELDS: *4 ounces*

½ cup distilled water

1 tablespoon loose leaf rooibos

1 tablespoon aloe vera juice

2 tablespoons Old-Fashioned Rosewater (see Chapter 7) or rose hydrosol

What you will need: teacup, strainer, 4-ounce bottle and cap or mister top, funnel

❶ To Make: Boil ½ cup distilled water and brew a small, strong cup of rooibos. Let the infusion steep for 15–20 minutes. Strain the herbs from the brew and place in the fridge and cool completely, 10–15 minutes. Once the brew has cooled, use the funnel to add the aloe vera juice and rosewater to the bottle. Top off with the rooibos brew. Cap tightly and shake well.

❷ To Store: Store in bottle and use within 1 month, or store in the refrigerator to extend the shelf life to 2–3 months.

❸ To Use: Use twice per day after cleansing. Moisten a cotton pad and gently sweep over facial skin to remove the last traces of dirt, oil, and makeup. Follow with moisturizer and serum.

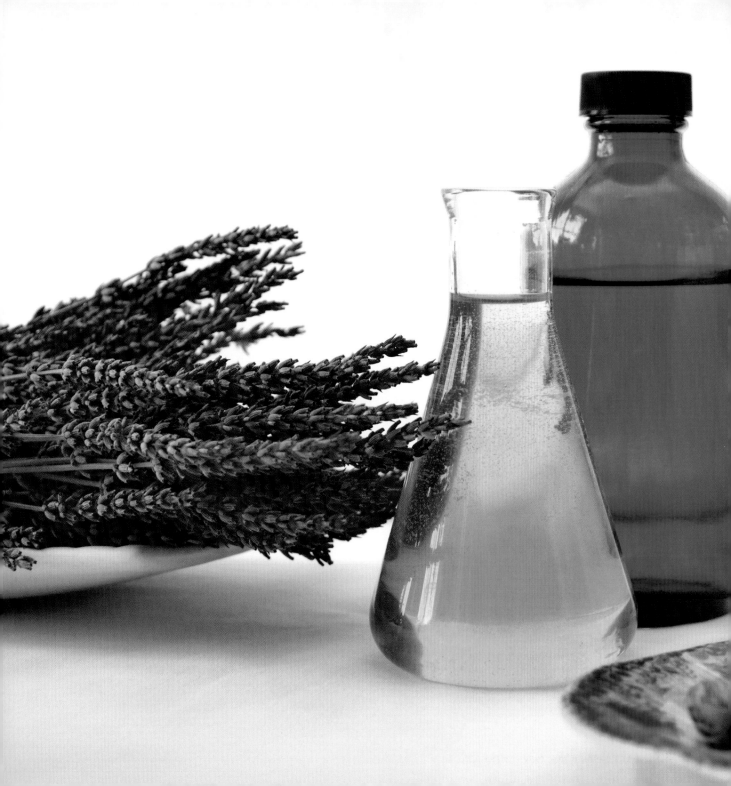

Balancing
FACIAL MOISTURIZER

This Balancing Facial Moisturizer is an ultra-light, ultra-nourishing astringent facial oil that will benefit people of all skin types, but especially those who have oily, acne-prone, or combination skin. The hazelnut oil, with deeply penetrating astringent properties, is highly beneficial for acne and helps to tone and tighten the skin. Grapeseed oil is ultra-light yet packed with nutrients and antioxidants that give skin a regenerative boost and a healthy glow. Both hazelnut and grapeseed oils are extremely high in vitamin E, which helps condition, repair, and protect your skin from premature aging due to exposure to UV rays and environmental pollutants. These luxurious botanical oils are complemented with an astringent, antibacterial, and reparative essential oil blend.

YIELDS: *1 ounce*

1 teaspoon Green Tea–Infused Oil
   (see Chapter 7)

2 teaspoons grapeseed oil

1 vitamin E capsule

4 drops tea tree essential oil

2 drops lemon essential oil

4 drops lavender essential oil

2 drops rosemary essential oil

3 teaspoons hazelnut oil

What you will need: dark-colored 1-ounce bottle with a dropper top, small funnel

❶ **To Make:** Place the funnel over your bottle and add the Green Tea–Infused Oil and grapeseed oil. Pierce the vitamin E capsule and squeeze the liquid out into the bottle, discarding the gel cap. Add the essential oils and fill up the bottle with hazelnut oil. Shake for a minute to blend.

❷ **To Store:** Store in bottle. Will keep for up to 6 months if stored out of direct sunlight.

❸ **To Use:** Use twice daily after cleansing and toning your skin. Facial oils work well on damp skin, so mist your skin with toner and apply a few drops of Balancing Facial Moisturizer to your fingertips. Emulsify the oil into the moisture on your skin from the mist. The added moisture will enable you to achieve an even application and help your skin absorb the beneficial botanicals deep into the dermal layers of your skin.

Vital
FACIAL MOISTURIZER

A richly moisturizing yet readily absorbed facial oil, this Vital Facial Moisturizer is perfect for dry, maturing, and environmentally damaged skin as well as sensitive and reactive skin types. It contains highly nutritious botanical oils that feed your skin the vitamins and nutrients it needs to fight premature aging. A veritable antioxidant powerhouse formulated to boost collagen production and condition, repair, and protect your skin, this moisturizer works hard to lessen the appearance and formation of fine lines and wrinkles.

YIELDS: *1 ounce*

1¾ teaspoon jojoba oil

1 teaspoon avocado oil

1¼ teaspoon grapeseed oil

2 vitamin E capsules

5 drops Australian sandalwood essential oil

5 drops rose geranium essential oil

2 drops patchouli essential oil

2 teaspoons Green Tea–Infused Oil (see Chapter 7)

What you will need: dark-colored 1-ounce bottle with a dropper top, small funnel

❶ **To Make:** Place the funnel over your bottle and add the jojoba, avocado, and grapeseed oils. Pierce the vitamin E capsules and squeeze the liquid out into the bottle, discarding the gel caps. Add the essential oils and fill up the bottle with Green Tea–Infused Oil. Shake for a minute to blend.

❷ **To Store:** Store in bottle. Will keep for up to 6 months if stored out of direct sunlight.

❸ **To Use:** Use twice daily after cleansing and toning your skin. Facial oils work well on damp skin, so mist your skin with toner and apply a few drops to your fingertips. Emulsify the oil into the moisture on your skin from the mist. The added moisture will enable you to achieve an even application and will help your skin absorb the beneficial botanicals deep into the dermal layers of your skin.

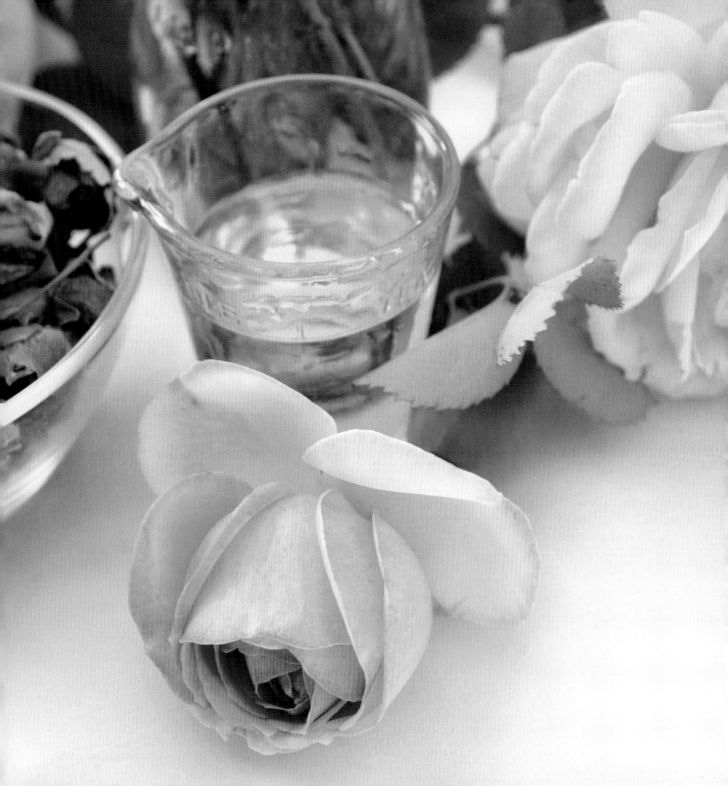

Luxurious
VITA-E FACIAL OIL

Silky and easily absorbed, this daily facial moisturizer is beneficial for all skin types, including sensitive and reactive skin. Grapeseed oil is ultra-light yet packed with nutrients and antioxidants, which give skin a regenerative boost and a healthy glow. With an exceptionally high vitamin E content, this moisturizer protects your skin cells from premature aging due to exposure to UV rays and environmental pollutants by effectively stopping free radical damage, promoting a healthy, glowing complexion.

YIELDS: *1 ounce*

2 teaspoons Green Tea–Infused Oil
(see Chapter 7)

1 teaspoon jojoba oil

2 vitamin E capsules

2 drops chamomile essential oil

3 drops rose geranium essential oil

6 drops lavender essential oil

3 teaspoons grapeseed oil

What you will need:
dark-colored 1-ounce bottle with a
dropper or pump top, small funnel

1 To Make: Place the funnel over your bottle and add the Green Tea–Infused Oil and jojoba oil. Pierce the vitamin E capsules and squeeze the liquid out into the bottle, discarding the gel caps. Add the essential oils and the grapeseed oil. Shake for a minute to blend.

2 To Store: Store in bottle. Will keep for up to 6 months if stored out of direct sunlight.

3 To Use: Use a few drops twice daily after cleansing and toning your skin. Facial oils work well on damp skin, so mist your skin with toner and apply a few drops to your fingertips. Emulsify the oil into the moisture on your skin from the mist. The added moisture will enable you to achieve an even application and help your skin absorb the beneficial botanicals deep into the dermal layers of your skin.

Green Tea
EYE CREAM

The active ingredients in this revitalizing under-eye cream help alleviate dark circles and puffy eyes while also reducing the appearance of fine lines and wrinkles. A little of this silky Green Tea Eye Cream will melt right into your skin for lovely results.

YIELDS: *½ ounce*

3 teaspoons Green Tea–Infused Oil (see Chapter 7)

2 vitamin E capsules

2 drops carrot seed essential oil

What you will need: boiling water, glass measuring cup, shallow bowl, chopstick, rubber spatula, jar with lid to hold ½ ounce of cream

1 **To Make:** Create a mini double boiler by pouring boiling water in the bottom of a shallow bowl. Put the Green Tea–Infused Oil into a glass measuring cup and place the cup into the bowl of boiling water to melt. Stir it a little to help it along. Once the oil has melted, remove the cup from the hot water and wipe dry. Pierce the vitamin E capsules and squeeze the liquid out into the melted oil, discarding the gel caps. Add the carrot seed essential oil and stir the ingredients together with a chopstick. Pour the melted oil into the jar and carefully put in the refrigerator. Remove after 30 minutes and screw the lid on tight. Label with contents and date.

2 **To Store:** Store in a cool dry place away from direct sunlight. Use within 1–1½ years.

3 **To Use:** Begin with clean skin. To use, remove a small amount of cream from the jar and melt between your fingertips. Then tap the cream onto the under-eye area and occipital bone.

SPA FACIAL STEAM
for Normal to Oily Skin

This Spa Facial Steam for Normal to Oily Skin works to soften your skin, open pores to loosen clogged debris, and release toxins.

YIELDS: *1 pint*

¾ cup dried comfrey

5 tablespoons dried lavender flowers

3 tablespoons dried rosemary

¼ cup dried parsley

¼ cup dried peppermint

¼ cup dried lemon peel

What you will need: mixing bowl, measuring cups, measuring spoons, 2 wooden spoons, pint-size canning jar with lid

1. **To Make:** Place all of the herbs in the mixing bowl and toss like a salad until you have a uniform blend. I like to use my hand to blend herbs, but you can also use 2 spoons. Transfer to the jar, label, and cap tightly.

2. **To Store:** Store in a cool dry place away from direct sunlight and use within 2 years.

3. **To Use:** To use, bring 4 cups of water to a boil, then remove from heat. Stir 2 tablespoons of the herbs into the water. Cover and let stand for 5 minutes. Carefully bring the pot to a table and make a tent over the pot with a bath towel to create a mini steam room. Clean your face, then hover over the steaming pot at least 8 inches away with your eyes closed. If the steam is too hot, open a vent to let some of the steam out and move your face a bit farther away from the steam. Breathe deeply, relaxing for 5–15 minutes. Note: If this whole production seems daunting, but you'd like the benefits of a facial steam, soak a washcloth in the herbal brew and place on your face for a few minutes, then repeat. Just be sure to let the cloth cool to a safe temperature before putting it on your skin. Note: Facial steams are not recommended for cystic acne, rosacea, or inflamed skin conditions.

Soothing
HERBAL STEAM

Sitting and breathing a lovely herbal facial steam sets the stage for a deeply relaxing and thoroughly cleansing home spa facial experience. Chamomile's sweet honey-apple aroma beautifully complements its soothing, regenerative properties. Relaxing lavender buds are an astringent, anti-inflammatory, and antibacterial herb. Rose is a healing, nourishing, and gentle astringent. Comfrey is soothing, healing, and anti-inflammatory. This recipe is beneficial for all skin types, especially dry, maturing, and sensitive.

YIELDS: *1 pint*

¼ cup dried **lavender flowers**

½ cup dried **chamomile flowers**

¾ cup dried **rose petals**

½ cup dried **comfrey leaves**

What you will need: mixing bowl, measuring cups, measuring spoons, 2 wooden spoons, pint-size canning jar with lid

① **To Make:** Place all of the herbs in the mixing bowl and toss like a salad until you have a uniform blend. I like to use my hand to blend herbs, but you can also use 2 spoons. Transfer to the jar, label, and cap tightly.

② **To Store:** Store jar in a cool dry place away from direct sunlight and use within 2 years.

③ **To Use:** To use, bring 4 cups of water to a boil, then remove from heat. Stir 2 tablespoons of the herbs into the water. Cover and let stand for 5 minutes. Carefully bring the pot to a table and make a tent over the pot with a bath towel to create a mini steam room. Clean your face, then hover over the steaming pot at least 8 inches away with your eyes closed. If the steam is too hot, open a vent to let some of the steam out and move your face a bit farther away from the steam. Breathe deeply, relaxing for 5–15 minutes. Note: If this whole production seems daunting, but you'd like the benefits of a facial steam, soak a washcloth in the herbal brew and place on your face for a few minutes, then repeat. Just be sure to let the cloth cool to a safe temperature before putting it on your skin. Note: Facial steams are not recommended for cystic acne or rosacea or inflamed skin conditions.

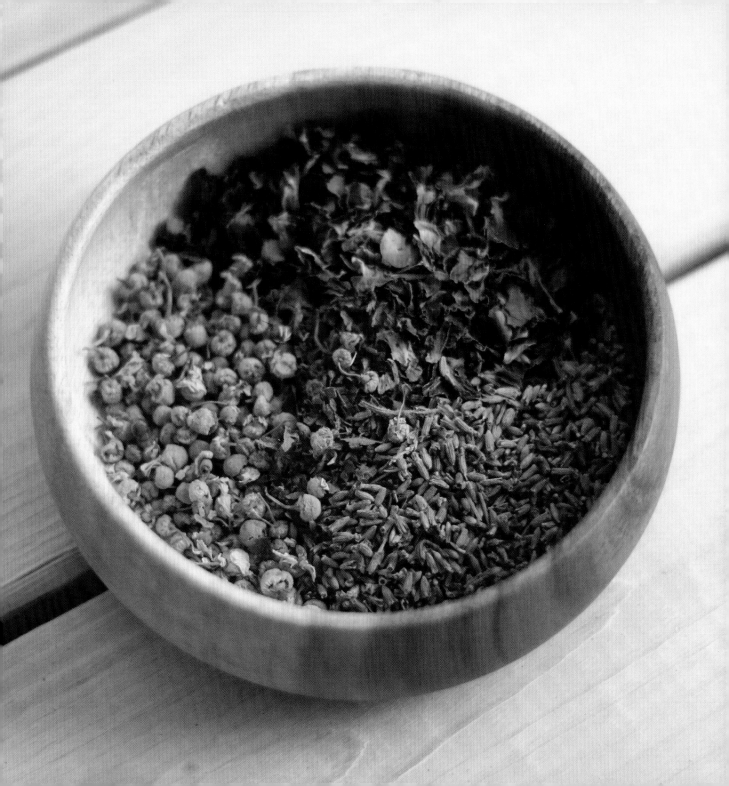

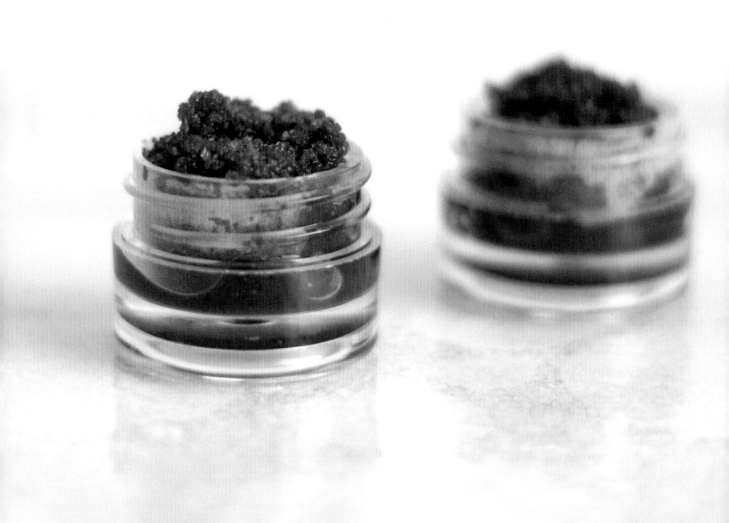

Chocolate
LIP SCRUB

Use this sensual lip smoother a couple times a week to help smooth out chapped lips. This intoxicatingly decadent lip scrub is completely edible as long as you use only food-grade ingredients, so use your favorite chocolate bar to make this recipe extra delectable. Needless to say, this one is great for Valentine's Day and makes a great gift too!

YIELDS: *2 ounces*

1 tablespoon coconut oil

½ teaspoon raw honey

½ teaspoon raw cocoa powder

¼ teaspoon vanilla extract

2 tablespoons fine granulated sugar

1 tablespoon grated chocolate

What you will need: measuring spoons, shallow mixing bowl, glass measuring cup, grater, fork, 2-ounce jar with lid

1 To Make: Create a mini double boiler by pouring boiling water in the bottom of a shallow bowl. Put the coconut oil into a glass measuring cup. Place the measuring cup into the bowl of hot water to melt and stir it a little to help it along. Once the oil is melted, remove the measuring cup from the hot water and wipe dry. Add the honey, cocoa powder, and vanilla and stir the ingredients together with a fork. Add the sugar and mix well. Grate the chocolate and stir it in.

2 To Store: To preserve the freshness of this natural scrub, do not get water into the jar. Label and store this scrub in a sealed jar in a cool dark place, out of direct sunlight, for up to a year.

3 To Use: Apply to your lips in small, circular motions. Massage with a light touch and rinse well. Use 1–2 times per week. Note: Do not use on severely chapped lips, split lips, or open wounds.

Green Tea and Adzuki
CLEANSING GRAINS

Traditional Asian facial cleansing grains, like this one, use adzuki beans that gently exfoliate without damaging the surface of the skin. In addition, green tea is a powerful antioxidant that helps rejuvenate the skin, prevent and repair sun damage, and promote elasticity. And the healing powers of chamomile calm and soothe redness and irritation.

YIELDS: *1 pint*

½ cup adzuki beans

½ cup green tea leaves

½ cup chamomile flowers

½ cup brown rice flour

½ cup kaolin clay

What you will need: face mask, coffee grinder, mixing bowl, fine-meshed sieve, pint-size canning jar with lid, spice jar with sifter cap (optional)

① **To Make:** Before you begin, find a protective face mask, or tie a bandana to cover your nose and mouth, to avoid breathing the powders. Next, put the adzuki beans, green tea, and chamomile into the jar, close the lid, and shake. Fill a coffee grinder with the mixture and grind to a very fine powder. Place the sieve over the mixing bowl. Empty the grinder into the sieve. Carefully sift the powder into the bowl. Put anything that doesn't sift through back into the grinder and leave the powder in the bowl. Fill the grinder with the adzuki, tea, and chamomile mixture. Repeat until all of the mix has been ground, discarding any woody bits that won't grind down. Next, sift the brown rice flour into the bowl and discard any larger rice grains. Carefully put the powders into the canning jar and add the kaolin clay. Close the lid tightly and shake well to blend to a uniform powder. Let stand for 5 minutes or so, letting the dust settle into the jar.

② **To Store:** Store this dry facial scrub in a spice jar with a sifter cap. To fill the jar, make a funnel by rolling up a piece of paper. Twist one end to open wide enough to fit into the spice jar, and the other wider to funnel in the powder. Tape it together and spoon the powder into the jar a little at a time. Once the jar is full, replace the sifter and cap, and this scrub is ready to use! You can also store this in the jar, using a clean dry spoon to dispense the cleansing grains. Keep the lid tightly closed when not in use and store for up to a year.

③ **To Use:** Simply tap out a bit of the powder into the palm of your hand and mix with water added a tiny bit at a time until a paste forms. Then softly cleanse your face using small circular motions. Rinse with warm water and follow with toner and moisturizer.

SKIN CARE SECRETS

For a more intensive facial treatment, make a replenishing facial mask by blending these cleansing grains with honey, yogurt, milk, rosewater, and/or toner and leave on for 5-20 minutes. Rinse with warm water to soften the mask and gently exfoliate your skin using small circular motions. Follow with toner and moisturizer.

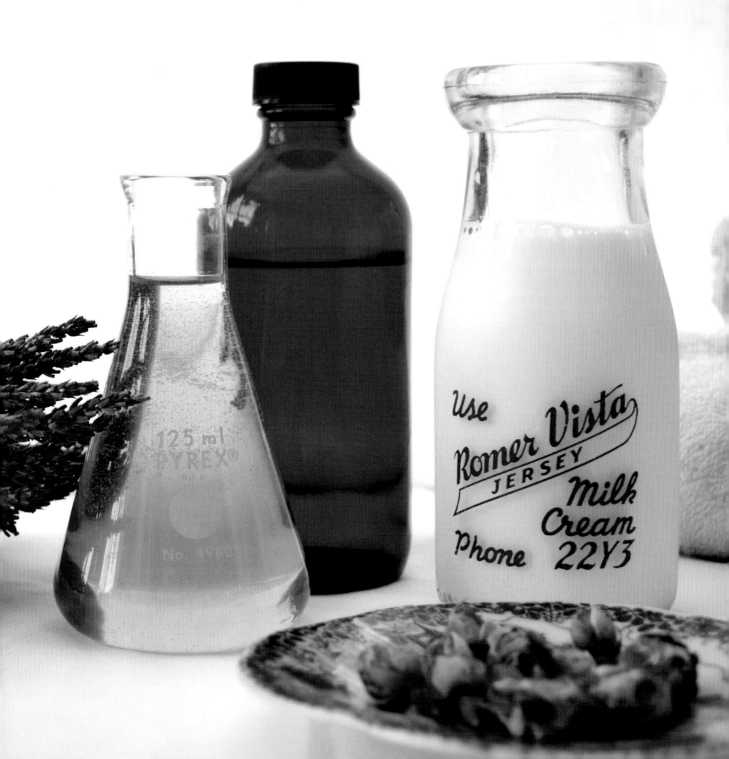

CHAPTER 3

FACIAL MASKS

The experience of relaxing with a facial mask on the skin is like no other. This is why most women you know will have at least a few different facial masks in their bathroom cabinet. The subtleties of temperature and texture excite the senses. Will the texture be smooth or gooey? Thick and rich like Carrot-Coconut NutraMoist Mask or light and refreshing like the Fresh Petals Mask? The scents waft over you and can carry you on a sensory journey over glorious earthen clay with the Green Clay Rose Milk Mask, a fresh glint of citrus with the Radiant Orange Mask, or a soothing waft of florals with the Agave Rose Anti-Aging Mask.

Enjoy the journey to beautiful skin as the treatment masks in this chapter improve your skin, visibly sucking the excess oil and toxins out of your pores or boosting your cells with vital nutrients and moisture. Removing the mask reveals fresh skin that's smoother, plumper, clearer, and more radiant than before. You'll be glowing from the inside, and your skin will radiate health and vitality. You are so beautiful!

Yerba Flax
FACE-FOOD MASK

Packed with nearly 200 beneficial bio-actives straight from the Amazon jungle, yerba mate packs a youthful punch in this superfood mask for radiant skin. Densely nutritious, this mask literally feeds your skin with beneficial moisture, reparative antioxidants, amino acids, vitamins, and minerals. Antibacterial honey increases circulation to help carry the nutrients into your skin cells to do their good work. Using this mask once per week promotes radiant vitality for all skin types, especially damaged, overexposed, and maturing skin.

YIELDS: *1–2 masks*

1 tablespoon loose-leaf yerba mate

⅛ cup water

1 tablespoon ground flax meal

1 teaspoon honey

½ teaspoon flaxseed oil

What you will need: coffee grinder, saucepan, mixing bowl, fork, tight-sealing storage container

1 **To Make:** Grind the yerba mate into a coarse powder in your coffee grinder. Boil the water in a saucepan. Place the yerba mate and flax meal in the mixing bowl and add the boiling water. Stir to moisten and let stand 5–10 minutes. Add the honey and flaxseed oil and blend with a fork to a uniform consistency. You will have a thick paste.

2 **To Store:** This mask is best fresh. Store in a closed container in the refrigerator and use within 4 days.

3 **To Use:** To use, spread a thick layer of the mask onto clean skin. Leave on skin 10–15 minutes and rinse off with warm water. Follow with toner and moisturizer.

Radiant Orange
MASK

Oranges are rich in vitamin C, which encourages collagen production and improves the elasticity of your skin. Agave is a natural antibacterial and humectant. Beneficial in lightening sunspots and acne scars, this invigorating Radiant Orange Mask works to unclog pores and improve circulation for a more radiant skin tone.

YIELDS: *1–2 masks*

1 teaspoon almond meal

1 teaspoon dried orange peel powder

1 teaspoon raw agave nectar

1½ teaspoons plain yogurt

What you will need: mixing bowl, spoon, tight-sealing storage container

❶ **To Make:** Place the almond meal and orange peel powder in a bowl. Add the agave nectar and yogurt and stir well to blend to a uniform consistency.

❷ **To Store:** This mask is best fresh. Store in a closed container in the refrigerator and use within 5 days.

❸ **To Use:** Spread a thick layer of the mask onto clean skin. Leave on skin 10–15 minutes and rinse off with warm water. Follow with toner and moisturizer.

HELPFUL HINTS

If you can't find orange peel powder, you can easily make it yourself! Start by peeling an orange. Cut the peel into smaller chunks and leave on a plate to air-dry for 24 hours or until completely dry. Grind the dried orange peel into a powder in a coffee grinder. Store in a tightly sealed container.

Green Clay
ROSE MILK MASK

Clay masks work wonders on the skin by soaking out excess oils and toxins and unclogging, clarifying, and refining pores for porcelain-soft skin. This recipe is designed so that you can make and store the dry portion ahead of time, mixing up a single-use fresh mask as desired by adding a little rosewater to make a spreadable paste. This mask is beneficial for oily, combination, normal, sensitive, congested, and acne-prone skin types.

YIELDS: *1 cup dry mask*

½ cup green clay

¼ cup kaolin clay

¼ cup powdered milk (full-fat dairy, soy, or coconut)

Rosewater

What you will need: face mask, small mixing bowl, spoon, 8-ounce jar and lid

❶ To Make: Before you begin, find a protective face mask, or tie a bandana to cover your nose and mouth, to avoid breathing the powders. Place the dry ingredients into the jar, place the lid on tightly, and shake to blend. Label with contents and date and store for up to a year. Right before you're ready to use the mask, mix 2 teaspoons powdered mixture with rosewater in a small bowl. Add the rosewater a little at a time, stirring to moisten all of the powder until you reach the desired consistency.

❷ To Store: Store the dry ingredients in an airtight container for up to 1 year. Once the dry ingredients are blended with the rosewater, store in a closed container in the refrigerator and use within 4 days.

❸ To Use: Spread a thick layer of the mask onto clean skin. Leave on skin 10–25 minutes and rinse off with warm water. Sensitive skin types should rinse off within 5–10 minutes. Follow with toner and moisturizer.

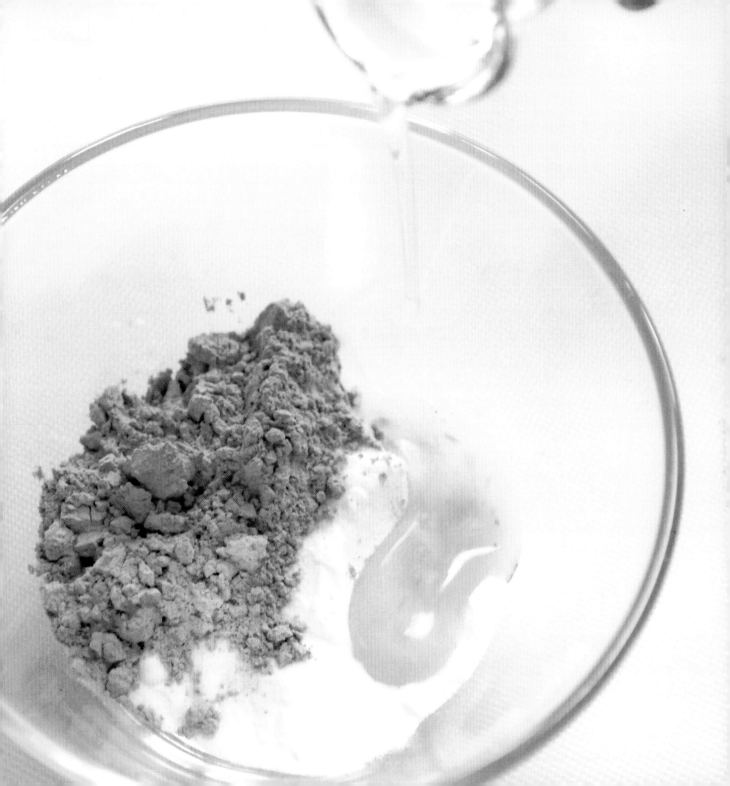

Clarifying
PROBIOTIC MOISTURE SURGE

This oil-based Clarifying Probiotic Moisture Surge cleans your skin with an anti-aging probiotic
burst of proteins. The jojoba oil, which is easily absorbed by your skin, delivers the potent antioxidants
of the green tea and the living probiotic nutrients deep into the dermal layers of your skin.
Your clogged pores are purged and your skin is left supple, alive, and positively glowing!

YIELDS: *1 mask*

4 probiotic capsules

**About 1 teaspoon Green Tea–Infused Oil
(see Chapter 7)**

1 drop chamomile essential oil

2 drops lavender essential oil

What you will need: small
bowl, spoon

1 **To Make:** Open the probiotic capsules and empty them into bowl,
discarding the empty capsules. Add the Green Tea–Infused Oil
a little at a time, stirring to moisten all of the powder until you reach
the desired consistency. Stir gently to blend, being careful not to breathe
the powder. Add essential oils and stir until blended.

2 **To Store:** This mask should not be stored. Use immediately.

3 **To Use:** Apply generously to clean skin. Gently massage the oil into
your skin using gentle upward strokes. You are essentially feeding your
face with phytonutrients, so take the few extra minutes to massage the
nutrients into your skin and relax those wrinkles. Use a feather-light
touch and the facial massage will help relax your wrinkles. Be mindful
not to stretch or pull at your facial skin, however. Leave on skin 10–25
minutes and rinse off with a steamy washcloth. Follow with toner and
moisturizer.

Carrot-Coconut

NUTRAMOIST MASK

Topically applied, carrots are known to stimulate cellular renewal, fortifying and repairing tissues, while they work to disarm free radicals, preventing premature aging. Packed with phytonutrients and beneficial moisture, this rejuvenating facial mask works to balance oil production and clarify pores for all skin types, especially dry, oily, and sensitive skin types.

YIELDS: *2–3 masks*

1 small carrot

2 teaspoons coconut oil

½ teaspoon coconut flour

1 teaspoon lemon juice, optional

What you will need: mixing bowl, fork, saucepan with lid and steamer, small tight-sealing storage container

1 **To Make:** Cut the carrot into chunks and place in a vegetable steamer. Steam on medium heat until soft enough to mash with a fork. Remove from heat. Place the carrot in your mixing bowl. Add the coconut oil and begin mashing them together. The coconut oil will melt with the heat of the carrot. Once well blended, add the coconut flour and blend to a uniform consistency. Add lemon juice if desired and stir well.

2 **To Store:** This mask is best fresh. Store in a closed container in the refrigerator and use within 4 days.

3 **To Use:** Spread a thick layer of the mask onto clean skin. Leave on skin 10 minutes and rinse off with warm water. Follow with toner and moisturizer. Use caution as carrot pulp may stain light-colored fabrics.

SKIN CARE SECRETS

Lemon juice adds additional astringent and lightening properties to this nourishing mask. Add the lemon juice if you have oily or combination skin.

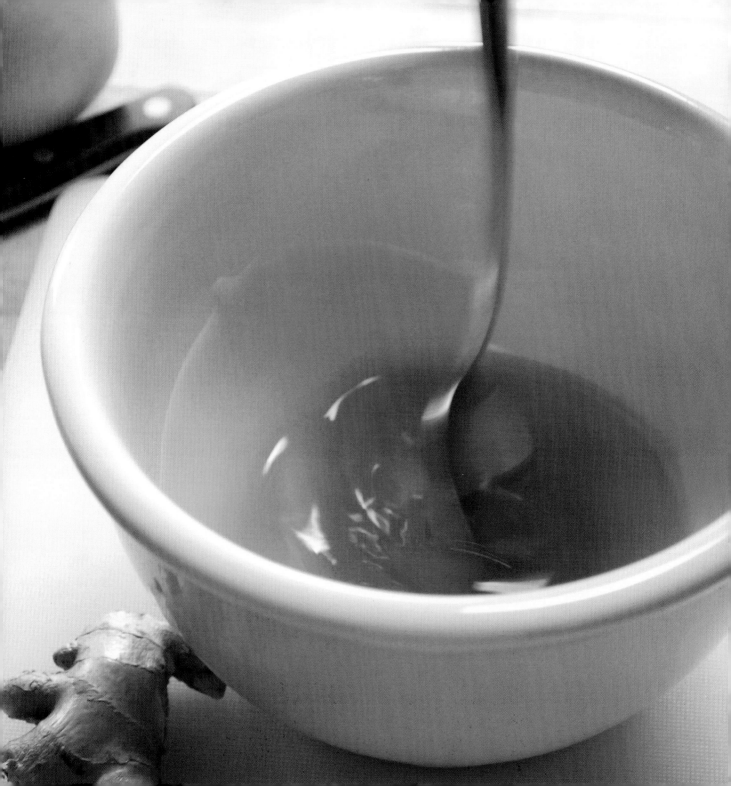

Aztec
HONEY AND WINE MASK

This quick and easy facial mask works to increase the radiance and vitality of your skin. Since ancient times, the tiny chia seeds found in this recipe were revered as superfoods by indigenous Central and South American peoples, including the Aztecs and Mayans, for their high levels of vital nutrients, omega-3 fatty acids, proteins, and antioxidants, and the red wine has exceptional levels of antioxidants known for their anti-aging benefits. In addition, the alcohol in the red wine tightens and clarifies pores while the honey hydrates and increases circulation.

YIELDS: *1 mask*

1 teaspoons raw honey
1½ teaspoons red wine
½ teaspoon ground chia seeds

What you will need:
small mixing bowl, fork

❶ To Make: Stir together the honey and red wine in a small mixing bowl. Add the ground chia seeds a little at a time, stirring with a fork to moisten all of the powder until you reach the desired consistency.

❷ To Store: This mask should not be stored. Use immediately.

❸ To Use: Spread a thick layer of the mask onto clean skin. Leave on skin 10–25 minutes and rinse off with warm water. Follow with toner and moisturizer.

Coco-Superfruit
MASK

This triple-berry blast of antioxidant superfruits rich in essential fatty acids helps nourish, soothe, and repair skin cells. These fruity antioxidants excel in scavenging free radicals and disarming them. Unchecked, free radicals attack and destroy your healthy cells. This mask is formulated to repair and regenerate while gently exfoliating for a fresh and radiant skin tone. This mask works wonders to improve environmentally damaged or maturing skin and is beneficial for normal, dry, oily, or combination skin types as well.

YIELDS: *1–2 masks*

1 strawberry

2 blueberries

1 raspberry

½ teaspoon raw honey

1 teaspoon coconut flour

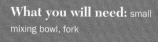

What you will need: small mixing bowl, fork

1 **To Make:** Place the berries in the mixing bowl and mash with the fork. Stir in the honey. Add the coconut flour a little at a time, stirring to moisten the powder until you have a thin, not drippy, spreadable paste. How much coconut flour you need will depend on how juicy your berries are. Coconut flour is highly absorbent, so start with a teaspoon and add more as needed, up to 3 teaspoons.

2 **To Store:** This mask should not be stored. Use immediately.

3 **To Use:** Spread a thick layer of the mask onto clean skin. Leave on skin 15–25 minutes and rinse off with warm water. Follow with toner and moisturizer. Use caution as the berries may stain light-colored fabrics.

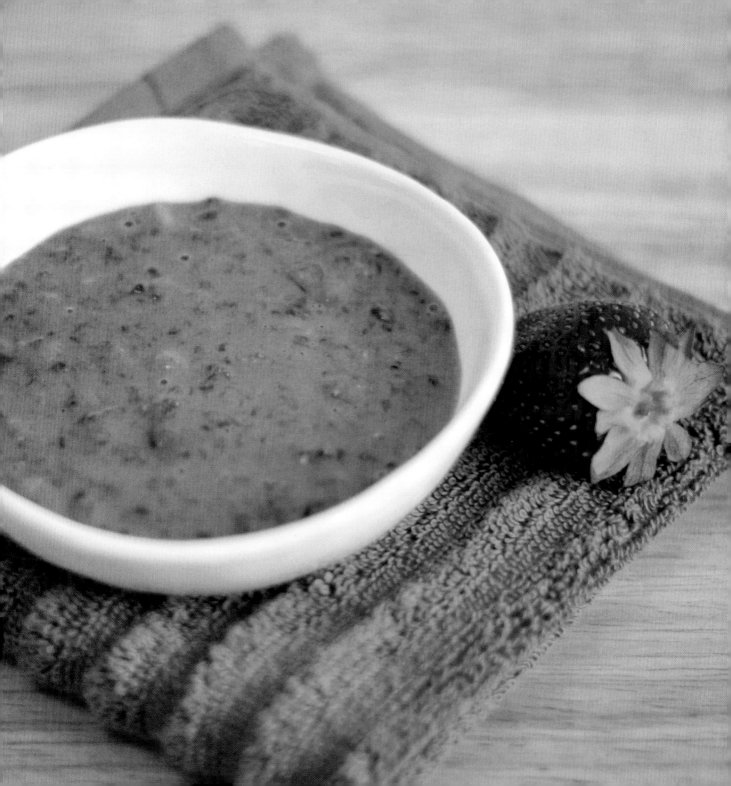

Chia Coconut
SUPERFOOD MASK

Amazing chia seeds are packed with vital nutrients, omega-3s, proteins, and antioxidants. In addition, the coconut found in this recipe is high in antioxidants and is hydrating and soothing for the skin. If you can, use fresh coconut water in this recipe and your skin will benefit from the naturally occurring electrolytes in this tropical elixir. This powerfully rejuvenating mask is also quite gentle and will benefit even the most sensitive of skin types.

YIELDS: *1–2 masks*

½ teaspoon chia seeds

1½ teaspoons coconut water

½ teaspoon coconut milk

What you will need: mixing bowl, fork, tight-sealing container

1. **To Make:** Place the chia seeds, coconut water, and coconut milk in the mixing bowl and stir with a fork. Soak the chia seeds for 5–10 minutes until all of the liquid has been absorbed and a gel has formed.

2. **To Store:** This mask is best fresh. Store in a closed container in the refrigerator and use within 4 days.

3. **To Use:** Spread a thick layer onto clean skin. Leave on skin 15–25 minutes and rinse off with warm water. Follow with toner and moisturizer.

Soothing
OIL-FREE MASK

Gain the hydrating, nourishing, and regenerative benefits of vitamin-rich flax without any added oil. This gentle, skin-tightening, moisturizing facial mask will soften and replenish all skin types.

YIELDS: *3–4 masks*

1 cup water

¼ cup flaxseeds

2 drops chamomile essential oil

What you will need: saucepan, wire whisk, mixing bowl, tea strainer, tight-sealing container

1. **To Make:** Place the water and flaxseeds in the pan on medium-high heat. Stir occasionally with the whisk to keep the seeds moving and not sticking to the pan. Once the mixture begins to boil, stir gently and constantly. When it starts to thicken slightly, turn down the heat to low and keep stirring until the seeds start suspending in the liquid instead of falling to the bottom of the pan. Remove from heat and strain liquid into the mixing bowl, discarding the seeds. Add the chamomile essential oil and whisk to blend. Allow to cool completely before use.

2. **To Store:** This mask is best fresh. Store in a closed container in the refrigerator for up to 1 week.

3. **To Use:** Spread a medium-thick layer of the mask onto clean skin. Leave on skin 10–15 minutes and rinse off with warm water. Follow with toner and moisturizer.

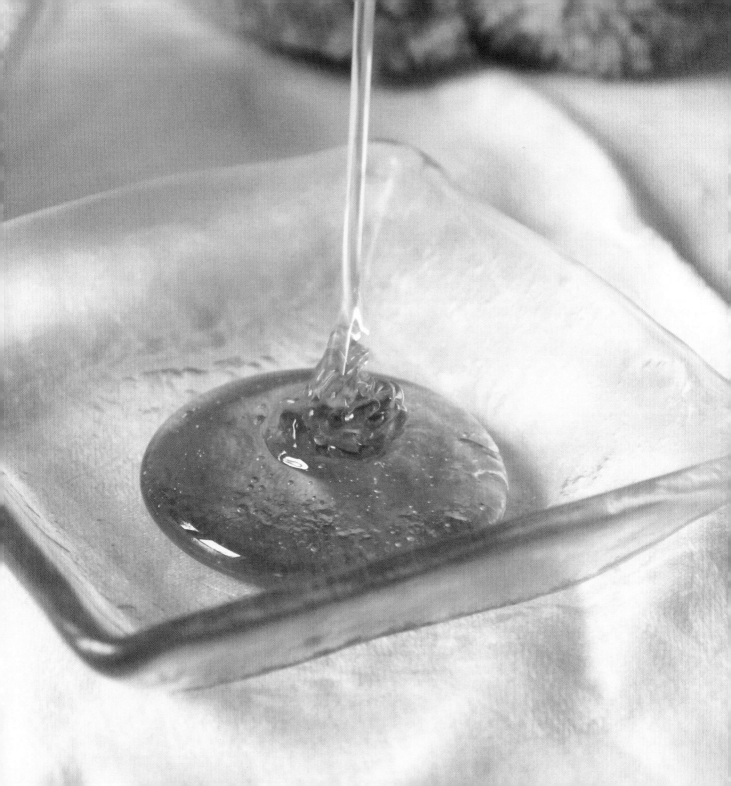

Manuka and Parsley
LIGHTENING ACNE MASK

Manuka honey is said to be the most beneficial for acne-prone skin due to its highly antibacterial nature, but it's okay to substitute regular honey if you can't find manuka. Parsley is rich in vitamins and nutrients and has skin-lightening properties, which help to fade acne scars and dark spots. This powerful herbal mask is beneficial for oily and acne-prone skin types. It can be used once per week.

YIELDS: *2–3 masks*

½ cup fresh flat-leaf parsley leaves

1 teaspoon lemon juice

1 tablespoon manuka honey

1–2 teaspoons kaolin clay

What you will need: blender, knife, cutting board, rubber spatula, small bowl, tight-sealing container

❶ **To Make:** Place the parsley, lemon juice, and honey in the blender. Blend on low speed until you have a uniform mixture. Remove from the blender with a rubber spatula and place into a mixing bowl. Add the clay a little at a time, stirring to blend until you reach a spreadable paste.

❷ **To Store:** This mask is best fresh. Store in a closed container in the refrigerator and use within 4 days.

❸ **To Use:** Apply to clean skin. Leave on skin 10–15 minutes and rinse off with warm water. You may experience a mild stinging sensation from the lemon juice. This is normal, especially if you have active acne blemishes. Rinse immediately if you experience discomfort. Follow with toner and moisturizer.

HELPFUL HINTS

I prefer to use flat-leaf parsley, which has a higher concentration of vital nutrients, in this recipe. If you can't find it, the curly leaf variety is a fine substitute.

Go Green
MOISTURE MASK

Go green with the avocado and spirulina found in this recipe and your skin will glow from the life-giving vitamins, emollients, and vital antioxidants in this super-nutrient-charged facial mask. Avocado is hydrating, nourishing, and regenerative, and every molecule in spirulina is skin food for a pure, natural healthy glow. This easy-to-make superfood moisturizing facial mask is beneficial for all skin types, especially dull, dry, and sensitive skin.

YIELDS: *1–2 masks*

½ **small avocado**

¼ **teaspoon lemon juice**

1 **teaspoon spirulina**

½ **teaspoon olive oil**

What you will need: mixing bowl, fork

❶ **To Make:** Scoop the avocado out of its shell and place into your mixing bowl. Add the lemon juice, spirulina, and olive oil. Mash the ingredients together with the back of your fork until you have a smooth, even consistency.

❷ **To Store:** This mask should not be stored. Use immediately.

❸ **To Use:** Spread a medium-thick layer of the mask onto clean skin. Leave on skin 10–20 minutes and rinse off with warm water. Follow with toner and moisturizer.

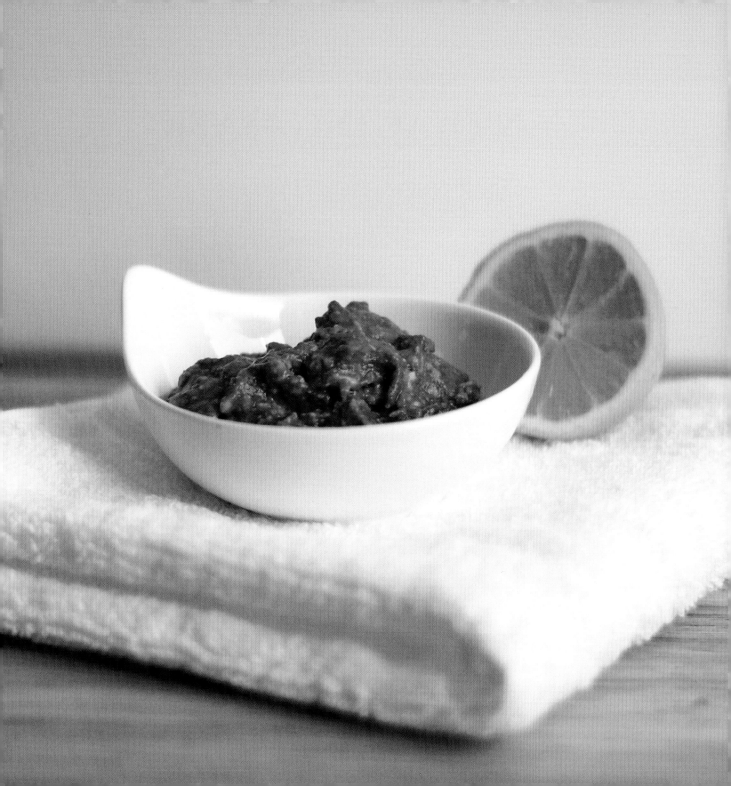

Agave Rose
ANTI-AGING MASK

The grapeseed oil found in this recipe contains the flavonoid oligomeric procyanidin, which is an amazingly strong antioxidant, about 50 times stronger than vitamins A and E. Grapeseed oil combined with soothing roses creates a magically healing, anti-inflammatory boost of botanical love for your skin. Hydrating and regenerative, this lovely soothing facial mask is beneficial for all skin types, especially maturing and sensitive skin.

YIELDS: *1–2 masks*

2 teaspoons rose petal powder

½ teaspoon grapeseed oil

¼ teaspoon agave syrup

½ teaspoon rosewater

What you will need: mixing bowl, spoon

1 **To Make:** Place the rose petal powder, grapeseed oil, and agave into the bowl and stir. Add the rosewater a little at a time, stirring to moisten all of the powder until you reach the consistency of a thick but spreadable paste.

2 **To Store:** This mask should not be stored. Use immediately.

3 **To Use:** Apply a thick layer of the mask onto clean skin. Leave on skin 10–25 minutes and rinse off with warm water. Follow with toner and moisturizer.

Rainforest ELIXIR MASK

The South American rainforest contains a plethora of superfoods and medicinal plants, including yerba mate, which contains 24 vitamins and minerals, 15 amino acids, and 11 polyphenols. Combine yerba mate with acai berries, which have 10 times more antioxidants than red grapes, and coconut milk, which contains the vitamins C, E, B_1, B_3, B_5, and B_6 as well as iron, selenium, calcium, magnesium, and phosphorus, and you'll find that this Rainforest Elixir Mask gives you much, much more than a multivitamin for your skin.

YIELDS: *2–3 masks*

2 tablespoons yerba mate leaves or 2 yerba mate tea bags

1 cup boiling water

2 teaspoons acai berry powder

1 teaspoon coconut flour

½ teaspoon coconut cream

What you will need: 1-cup glass measuring cup, tea strainer, mixing bowl, spoon

❶ To Make: Place the yerba mate in the measuring cup and pour in the boiling water. Cover and let steep for 20 minutes or more. Strain out the yerba mate leaves and discard, reserving the brew. Place the acai powder, coconut flour, and coconut cream into the bowl and stir. Be mindful not to breathe the powders as you work with them. Add the brewed yerba mate a little at a time, stirring to moisten all of the powder until you reach the desired consistency of a thick but spreadable paste. You will use 1–2 teaspoons of brew.

❷ To Store: This mask is best fresh. Use immediately.

❸ To Use: Apply a thick layer of the mask onto clean skin. Leave on skin 10–25 minutes and rinse off with warm water. Follow with toner and moisturizer.

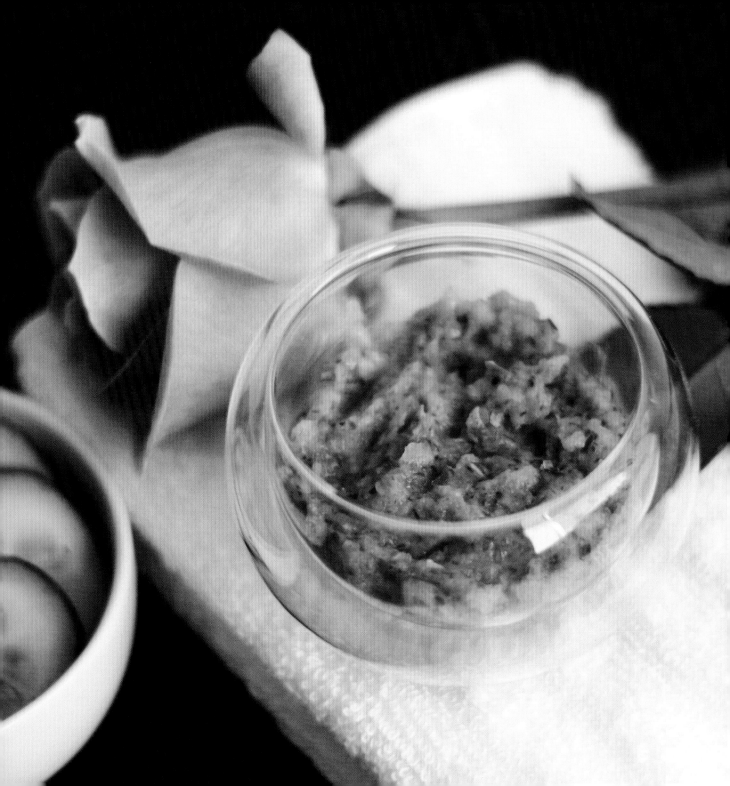

Fresh Petals MASK

Cucumbers and roses are widely known for their soothing, healing, and anti-inflammatory effects on the skin. This soothing, refreshing combination of cucumber and roses is beneficial for all skin types and conditions, especially sensitive, maturing, overexposed, sun-damaged, dry, or easily irritated skin.

YIELDS: *2–3 masks*

½ small cucumber

½ cup fresh rose petals

1 teaspoon Fresh Comfrey Oil (see Chapter 7), grapeseed oil, or your favorite carrier oil

What you will need: blender, knife, cutting board

❶ **To Make:** Cut the cucumber into chunks, discarding any excess water, leaving the pulp to make ¼ cup, and place into the blender. Next, add the rose petals to the blender and cover. Blend in short bursts on high, adding the comfrey oil a little at a time to achieve a thicker but uniform purée. Be careful not to overblend, as the mixture may liquefy.

❷ **To Store:** This mask is best fresh. Use immediately.

❸ **To Use:** Apply a thick layer of the mask onto clean skin. Leave on skin 10–30 minutes and rinse off with warm water. Follow with toner and moisturizer.

HELPFUL HINTS

Choose robustly blooming roses to pluck the petals from for this recipe. Pick them from your garden midmorning, after the dew has dried but before they wilt with the heat of the day. Remove the petals directly after cutting from the plant to preserve the highest nutrient value and reserve.

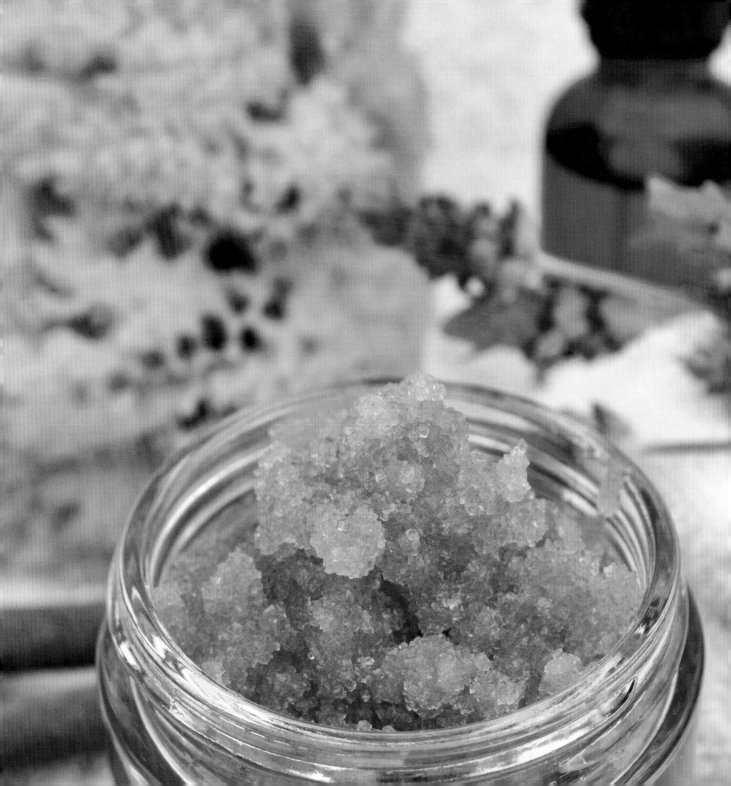

CHAPTER 4

BODY SCRUBS AND WASHES

A large part of the human experience is the act of bathing, becoming clean again. We shower to invigorate, to wake up and face the day. We wash off the day's work or play. We wash to primp and preen ourselves for social events. And we have learned to create little slices of sensory heaven within this daily experience by bringing scent, texture, and luxury to the bath and shower by using body washes and body scrubs that combine soap, exfoliant, and moisturizer into one amazing product.

In these recipes, a wide variety of nutritious exfoliating ingredients are combined with luxurious botanical oils and bioactive essential oils for aromatherapy benefits to the mind, body, and spirit. After all, who wants to wash with just soap when you can use a decadent body scrub like the Lemon Poppy Seed Scrub or a luxurious body wash like the Honey Coconut Body Wash? The unique body scrubs and washes included in this chapter are guaranteed to turn an ordinary shower into an extraordinary home spa experience!

Olive Butter SCRUB

The Castile soap used in this recipe balances the ultra-rich shea butter, leaving your skin moisturized but not oily. The addition of Castile creates a more emulsifying-type formula that rinses slightly cleaner than most typical oil-based scrubs. You will enjoy fresh, glowing skin with this clean, luxuriant moisturizing formula.

YIELDS: *20 ounces*

¾ cup shea butter

½ cup olive oil

¼ cup liquid Castile soap (unscented or lavender)

4 vitamin E capsules

30 drops lavender essential oil

30 drops lemon essential oil

1 cup fine-grained sea salt

What you will need: double boiler, rubber spatula, mixing bowl, measuring cups, fork, jars and lids to fit 20 ounces of scrub

1 To Make: Start the double boiler on medium heat. Once it reaches a boil, reduce heat to simmer. Place the shea butter in the top of the double boiler and cover. Simmer until melted, stirring occasionally. To preserve the beneficial botanicals, do not overheat. Once melted, remove from heat, take the top pan off the double boiler, and cool 5 minutes. Pour the melted shea butter into the mixing bowl, using the rubber spatula to get the remainder out of the pan. Add the olive oil and Castile soap. Pierce the vitamin E capsules and squeeze the liquid into the bowl, discarding the gel caps. Add the essential oils and stir well. Add the sea salt and blend to a uniform consistency. Spoon the mix into the jar or jars. Label with contents and date and seal tightly. The scrub is ready to use; however, the shea butter will continue to solidify the scrub as it cools over the next hour or so.

2 To Store: To preserve the freshness of this natural scrub, do not get water into the jar. Store this scrub in a sealed jar in a cool dark place, out of direct sunlight. Use up within 6 months to a year.

3 To Use: Use in place of a soap or body wash in your shower or bath. Apply to your skin in small, upward, circular motions. Massage the scrub in small circular motions, starting with the legs and arms, making your way up to the torso, ending at your heart. Rinse well.

Javanese Gold BODY SCRUB

Give your skin the royal treatment with this exotic botanical scrub high in beneficial emollients and antioxidants. Massage your skin with this modern version of Javanese Lulur, a royal traditional body treatment that dates back to the 17th century. The complete ritual starts with a full body massage, exfoliating scrub, and a bath scented with jasmine and roses, which is followed with a jasmine-infused moisturizer. The ladies of the family treat the bride-to-be with this decadent ritual every day for 40 days before her wedding ceremony. Enjoy the bliss of this exotic luxury—and the silky soft and glowing skin that comes with it—in your own home spa!

YIELDS: *21 ounces*

¼ cup extra-virgin coconut oil

½ cup sweet almond oil

3 tablespoons honey

1 tablespoon sesame seeds

1 cup turbinado sugar

½ cup brown rice flour

2 teaspoons turmeric

What you will need: blender, rubber spatula, mixing bowl, measuring cups, fork, jars and lids to fit 21 ounces of scrub

❶ To Make: Place the coconut oil, sweet almond oil, honey, and sesame seeds into the blender. Blend until you have a creamy, uniform consistency. The sesame seeds will retain some texture. Using the rubber spatula, scrape the mixture into the mixing bowl. Add the turbinado sugar, brown rice flour, and turmeric, blending the ingredients together with a fork until well mixed.

❷ To Store: Store this scrub in a sealed container in the refrigerator and use up within 3 months.

❸ To Use: Apply to damp skin in small, upward, circular motions. Take the extra time to give yourself a nice massage while applying the scrub. Start with the legs and arms and make your way up to the torso, ending at your heart. Rinse well. For added benefit, leave on your skin for an additional 10–20 minutes before rinsing off.

SKIN CARE SECRETS

You don't usually need any additional moisturizer after using a body scrub, and your skin is left very soft and radiantly healthy.

Sugar Chai
HONEY SCRUB

The exotic body scrub is made extra special with the use of the Chai Spice–Infused Oil. The warming, antioxidant-rich chai spices include cinnamon, cardamom, nutmeg, star anise, ginger, fennel, and black pepper. The black tea found in chai is beneficial in a body scrub formula, as the caffeine stimulates circulation, aids detoxification, and reduces the appearance of cellulite. In Ayurvedic traditions, chai spices are known to be calming, vitalizing, and mentally clarifying.

YIELDS: *20 ounces*

½ cup Chai Spice–Infused Oil (see Chapter 7)

¼ cup sweet almond oil, or favorite carrier oil

⅛ teaspoon ground cinnamon

⅛ teaspoon ground nutmeg

⅛ teaspoon ground cardamom

⅛ teaspoon ground ginger (dried, not fresh)

½ cup raw unpasteurized honey

½ cup almond meal

¾ cup brown sugar

What you will need: medium-size mixing bowl, measuring cups, fork, jars and lids to fit 20 ounces of scrub

1. **To Make:** In a medium-size mixing bowl, mix oils, spices, and honey with a fork until well blended. Stir in almond meal, mixing until blended. Then stir in brown sugar until you have a consistent texture.

2. **To Store:** To preserve the freshness of this natural scrub, do not get water into the jar. Store this scrub in a sealed jar in a cool dark place, out of direct sunlight. Use up within a year.

3. **To Use:** Use in place of a soap or body wash in your shower or bath. Apply to your skin in small, upward, circular motions. Massage the scrub in small circular motions, starting with the legs and arms, making your way up to the torso, ending at your heart. Rinse well.

HELPFUL HINTS

You can substitute ½ teaspoon fresh grated ginger for the dried ginger, but this will reduce the shelf life to 2 weeks, stored in the fridge.

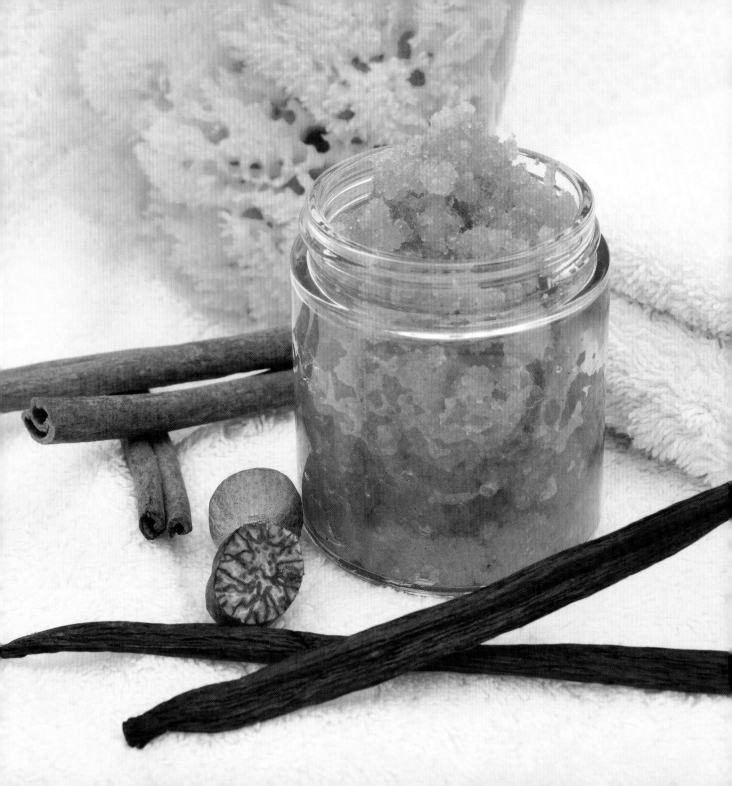

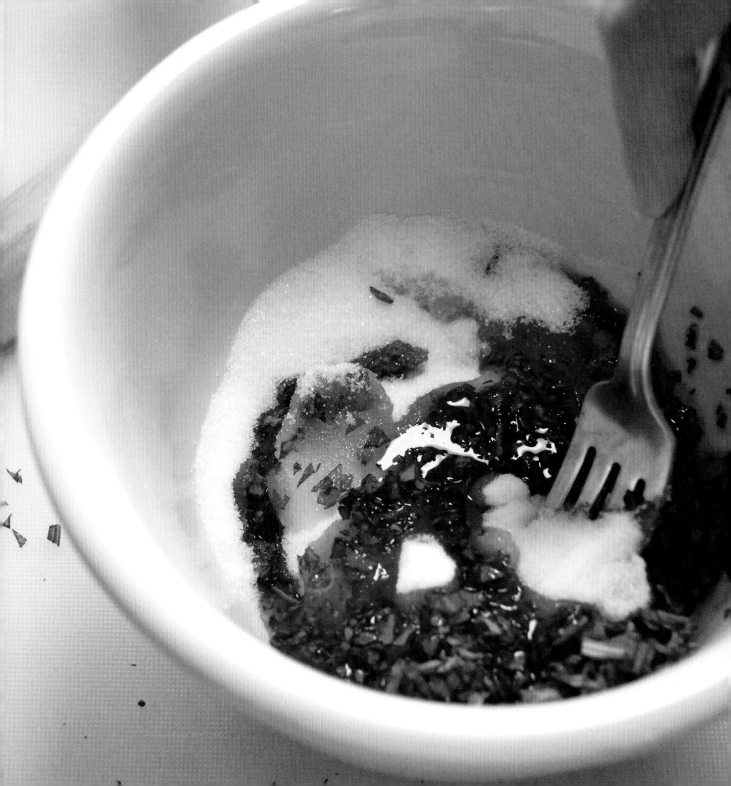

Herb Garden BODY SCRUB

Fresh garden herbs are a real treat for your skin. They are chock full of vitamins and nutrients that carry a multitude of skin care and aromatherapy benefits. For this recipe you can use any culinary herbs or flowers you have on hand, such as rosemary, parsley, basil, sage, rose petals, lavender flowers, and others. Pick them fresh from your garden or use what you have in the fridge! In addition, sea salts gently slough off dull, dry, dead skin while re-mineralizing your system, plus they help preserve the fresh herbs for a longer shelf life for this scrub.

YIELDS: *16 ounces*

½ cup freshly chopped herbs

1 cup sea salt

½ cup extra-virgin olive oil

What you will need: cutting board, knife, small mixing bowl, measuring cups, fork, jars and lids to fit 16 ounces of scrub

1 **To Make:** Place the chopped herbs, salt, and oil into a small mixing bowl. Blend the ingredients together with a fork until you have a uniform consistency.

2 **To Store:** Store this scrub in a sealed container in the refrigerator and use up within 3–4 weeks.

3 **To Use:** Use in place of a soap or body wash in your shower or bath. Apply to your skin in small, upward, circular motions. Massage the scrub in small circular motions, starting with the legs and arms, making your way up to the torso, ending at your heart. Rinse well.

HELPFUL HINTS

This scrub has a vibrant herbal scent due to the high levels of vital plant essences that the fresh herbs contain. Choose your fresh herbs and begin by washing and thoroughly air-drying them. Then pick the leaves, discarding the woody stems, and finely chop them for a soft aromatic exfoliation.

Gentle OATMEAL WASH

This simple botanical wash can be used daily in place of regular soap. The soothing, gentle oats and chamomile are excellent for sensitive skin or skin conditions such as eczema or psoriasis. You will be surprised how gorgeous this simple recipe is and how soft your skin will be afterwards. This soothing formula has a lovely and light natural unisex scent.

YIELDS: *24 ounces*

1 cup whole oats

1 bar moisturizing soap

1 cup chamomile flowers

½ cup powdered milk (soy, coconut, or dairy), optional

What you will need: cutting board, knife, grater, mixing bowl, measuring cups, wooden spoon (optional), jar, small muslin drawstring bag, three 8-ounce jars with lids

1. **To Make:** Coarsely chop the oats and put into the mixing bowl. Coarsely grate the soap and add to the bowl along with the chamomile. It's okay if the soap is a little gooey; just take care to break up any chunks, blending it in evenly with the other ingredients. Add the powdered milk if you desire a more moisturizing body wash. Feel free to mix this with your hands, or you can use a wooden spoon.

2. **To Store:** Put the mix in your jars and close the lids tightly. Label with contents and expiration date of 2 years. Store in a cool dry place away from direct sunlight. The filled herbal bag may be good for more than one bath if you store it in the freezer and thaw it out before your next bath or shower. To thaw, toss in the tub or soak for a few minutes in hot water.

3. **To Use:** Loosely fill the cloth bag with the mixture and tie a bow tight enough that it won't come apart in use. Remember, you will need to untie it later to clean out and use again. Use in place of a soap or body wash in your shower or bath. The herbal bag functions like a washcloth, but think of it as a teabag. Bring the herb-filled cloth bag into the shower or bath. Wet the bag well and slowly rub over your body with a gentle scrubbing motion. If in the bath, let the bag steep in the water as you bathe. Continue re-wetting the bag, squeezing the fragrant herbal elixir out over your body.

Mocha Latte SCRUB

Start your day with a vibrant and healthy glow when you use this yummy Mocha Latte Scrub. Coffee and chocolate contain regenerative antioxidants and naturally occurring caffeine, which increases circulation, while coffee grounds have a gritty but soft texture that works to promote ultra-smooth skin. This scrub is also a fantastic cellulite buster.

YIELDS: *16 ounces*

¼ cup finely ground coffee

½ cup raw sugar

1 tablespoon cocoa powder

1 tablespoon powdered milk (soy, coconut, or dairy)

1 cup sweet almond oil

4 vitamin E capsules

What you will need: rubber spatula, medium-size mixing bowl, measuring cups, fork, jars and lids to fit 16 ounces

1 **To Make:** Place the coffee, sugar, cocoa, and powdered milk in a medium-size mixing bowl. Add the oil and mix together with a fork until you have a uniform consistency. Pierce the vitamin E capsules and squeeze the liquid out into the bowl, discarding the gel caps. Stir well to blend.

2 **To Store:** To preserve the freshness of this natural scrub, do not get water into the jar. Store this scrub in a sealed jar in a cool dark place, out of direct sunlight. Use up within 6 months to a year.

3 **To Use:** Use in place of a soap or body wash in your shower or bath. Apply to your skin in small, upward motions. Massage the scrub in small circular motions, starting with the legs and arms, making your way up to the torso, ending at your heart. Rinse well.

HELPFUL HINTS

This body scrub is designed to leave beneficial oils on your skin; however, the cocoa powder may stick in your pores. If that is the case, wash with a mild soap and moisturize as desired.

Citrus Blast BODY SCRUB

Citrus fruits are high in vitamin C, which benefits your skin in amazing ways! Citrus contains naturally occurring alpha-hydroxy acids, which are known to have lightening effects on the skin. When topically applied, vitamin C enhances the production of collagen and boosts elasticity, helping your skin retain a firm and youthful appearance. In addition, using this Citrus Blast Body Scrub will help reduce the appearance of cellulite. It's a win-win!

YIELDS: *11 ounces*

Zest of ½ lemon

Zest of ½ lime

Zest of ½ orange

1 teaspoon fresh lemon juice

1 teaspoon fresh lime juice

1 teaspoon fresh orange juice

1 cup sea salt

¼ cup grapeseed oil

What you will need: grater, cutting board, knife, mixing bowl, measuring cups, fork, jars and lids to fit 11 ounces of scrub

1 **To Make:** Start with washing and thoroughly air-drying the citrus fruits. The fruit will be easier to work with if you leave it whole for removing the zest. Place the citrus zest and juices into the bowl. Add sea salt and grapeseed oil and blend the ingredients together with a fork until you have a uniform consistency.

2 **To Store:** Store this scrub in a sealed container in the refrigerator and use up within a week.

3 **To Use:** Use in place of a soap or body wash in your shower or bath. Apply to your skin in small, upward, circular motions. Massage the scrub in small circular motions, starting with the legs and arms, making your way up to the torso, ending at your heart. Rinse well.

SKIN CARE SECRETS

Citrus is known to increase your sensitivity to the sun, so it is best not to use this directly before sunbathing. Wear a sunscreen such as the Sun Protection Lotion Stick (see Chapter 9) and protective clothing if you go into the sun.

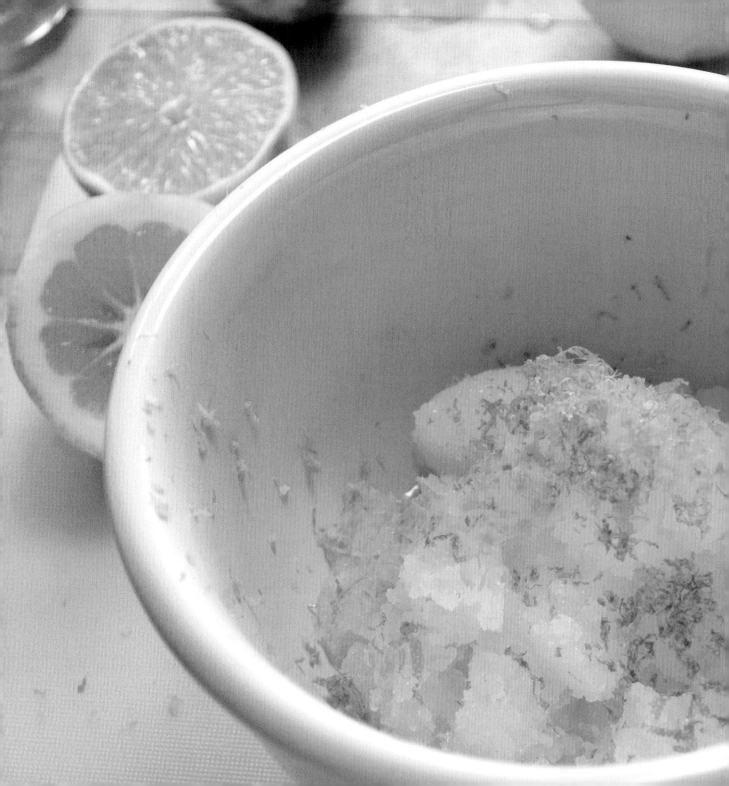

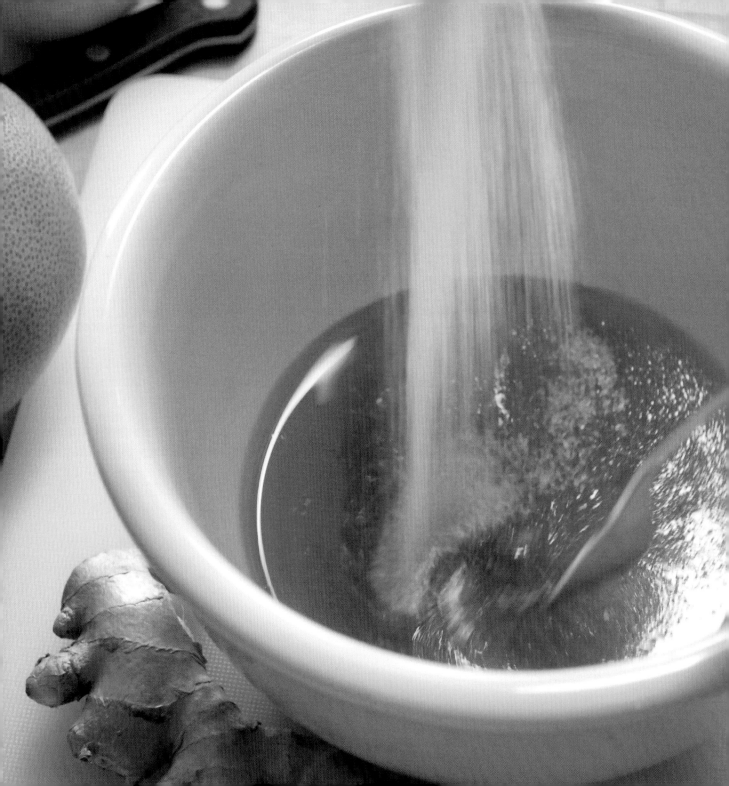

Vanilla, Bourbon, and Honey
SCRUB

The intoxicatingly decadent body scrub is made extra special
with the Vanilla-Infused Oil from Chapter 7.

YIELDS: *about 18 ounces*

½ cup Vanilla-Infused Oil

½ cup raw unpasteurized honey

1½ cups turbinado sugar

1 teaspoon bourbon

1 teaspoon vanilla extract

What you will need: medium-size mixing bowl, measuring cups, fork, jars and lids to fit 18 ounces of scrub

❶ **To Make:** In a medium-size mixing bowl, blend together the oil and honey. Mix them with a fork until you have a uniform consistency. Next, add the turbinado sugar and blend until you have a consistent texture. Stir in the bourbon and vanilla extract and it's ready to use!

❷ **To Store:** To preserve the freshness of this natural scrub, do not get water into the jar. Store this scrub in a sealed jar in a cool dark place, out of direct sunlight. Label with contents and expiration date of 1 year.

❸ **To Use:** Use in place of a soap or body wash in your shower or bath. Apply to your skin in small, upward, circular motions. Massage the scrub in small circular motions, starting with the legs and arms, making your way up to the torso, ending at your heart. Rinse well.

Almond
MOISTURE SCRUB

This yummy, buttery scrub is simply fabulous. The almond meal is both exfoliating and moisturizing and brings a unique soft texture to this body buffer. The addition of the shea butter to the recipe adds an extra-luxurious moisture boost. Since shea butter is a richer emollient than liquid carrier oils, such as sweet almond or grapeseed oils, this scrub will leave a richer, more moisturizing layer of beneficial oils on your skin. Scent this scrub with your favorite essential oil blend or leave unscented for a rich and buttery treat for your dry skin.

YIELDS: *18 ounces*

½ cup shea butter

½ cup sweet almond oil

4 vitamin E capsules

Essential oil blend
  (see Appendix A), optional

½ cup almond meal

¾ cup granulated sugar

What you will need: double boiler, rubber spatula, mixing bowl, measuring cups, fork, jars and lids to fit 18 ounces of scrub

① **To Make:** Start the double boiler on medium heat. Once it reaches a boil, reduce heat to simmer. Place the shea butter in the top of the double boiler and cover. Simmer until melted, stirring occasionally. To preserve the beneficial botanicals, do not overheat. Remove from heat, take the top pan off the double boiler, and cool 5 minutes. Pour the melted shea butter into the mixing bowl, using the rubber spatula to get the remainder out of the pan. Add the sweet almond oil. Pierce the vitamin E capsules and squeeze the liquid out into the melted shea butter, discarding the gel caps. If you are scenting the scrub, add the essential oils and stir. Add the almond meal and sugar, stirring to a uniform consistency. The scrub is ready to use; however, the shea butter will continue to solidify the scrub as it cools over the next hour or so.

② **To Store:** Spoon the mix into the jars. Label with contents and date and seal tightly. To preserve the freshness of this natural scrub, do not get water into the jar. Store this scrub in a sealed jar in a cool dark place, out of direct sunlight. Use up within 6 months to a year.

③ **To Use:** Use in place of a soap or body wash in your shower or bath. This is a thicker scrub due to the shea butter and may need to be softened or emulsified with a little water in your palm to make a spreadable scrub. Apply to your skin in small, upward, circular motions. Massage the scrub in small circular motions, starting with the legs and arms, making your way up to the torso, ending at your heart. Rinse well.

HELPFUL HINTS

You can substitute one of the infused oils from Chapter 7 for the sweet almond oil for added scent and therapeutic benefits.

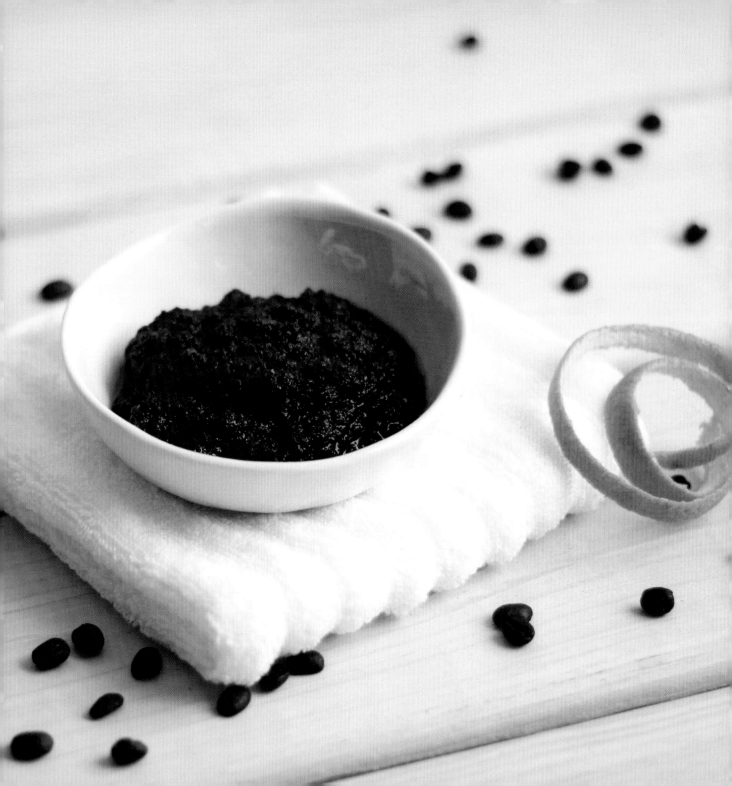

Valencia Coffee SCRUB

The natural caffeine in the coffee used in this recipe boosts circulation and works to effectively reduce the appearance of cellulite. Oranges stimulate new cell production, promoting increased collagen levels, encouraging firm skin. Enjoy this fresh and flirty orange-infused coffee scrub, an aromatic combination that benefits your mind, body, and spirit.

YIELDS: *about 15 ounces*

¼ cup finely ground coffee

1 cup turbinado sugar

Zest of 1 orange

⅔ cup olive oil

15 drops Sweet Citrus Essential Oil (Appendix A)

What you will need: medium-size mixing bowl, measuring cups, fork, jars and lids to fit 15 ounces of scrub

❶ **To Make:** Place the coffee, sugar, and orange zest in a medium-size mixing bowl. Add the olive oil and essential oil and mix together with a fork until you have a uniform consistency.

❷ **To Store:** To preserve the freshness of this natural scrub, keep water out of it. Store this scrub in a sealed container and use up within 6 months.

❸ **To Use:** Use in place of a soap or body wash in your shower or bath. Apply to damp skin in small, upward motions. Massage the scrub in small circular motions, starting with the legs and arms, making your way up to the torso, ending at your heart. Rinse well.

SKIN CARE SECRETS

Body scrubs are designed to exfoliate away dead skin cells and leave nourishing scented oils on your skin. For maximum benefit, do not use soap to wash off these residual oils. Towel off and the nutrients in the botanical oils will greatly benefit your skin, soaking in after a few minutes.

Floral

OATMEAL WASH

This simple botanical wash can be used daily in place of soap. This batch is large enough to share with friends and family. Have fun picking out decorative jars and adorning them with painted flowers or a cute label. Tie a ribbon around the jars or paint the lids a pretty color. Clear glass allows you to see how lovely the finished product is.

YIELDS: *24 ounces*

1 cup whole oats

1 bar moisturizing soap

⅓ cup dried chamomile flowers

⅓ cup dried rose petals

⅓ cup dried lavender flowers

½ cup powdered milk (soy, coconut, or dairy), optional

What you will need: cutting board, knife, grater, mixing bowl, measuring cups, spoon, jar, small muslin drawstring bag, three 8-ounce jars with lids

❶ **To Make:** Coarsely chop the oats and put into the mixing bowl. Coarsely grate the soap and add to the bowl along with the chamomile, rose petals, and lavender. Add the powdered milk if you desire a more moisturizing body wash. It's okay if the soap is a little gooey; just take care to break up any chunks, blending them in evenly with the other ingredients. Feel free to mix this with your hands, or use a wooden spoon.

❷ **To Store:** Put the Floral Oatmeal Wash in your jars and close the lids tightly. Label with contents and expiration date of 2 years. Store in a cool dry place away from direct sunlight. The filled herbal bag may be good for more than one bath if you store it in the freezer and thaw it out before your next bath or shower. To thaw, toss in the tub or soak for a few minutes in hot water.

3 **To Use:** Loosely fill the cloth bag with the Floral Oatmeal Wash. Tie a bow tight enough that it won't come apart in use. Remember, you will need to untie it later to clean out and use again. Use in place of a soap or body wash in your shower or bath. The herbal bag functions like a washcloth, but think of it as a teabag. Bring the herb-filled cloth bag into the shower or bath. Wet the bag well and slowly rub over your body with a gentle scrubbing motion. If in the bath, let the bag steep in the water as you bathe. Continue re-wetting the bag, squeezing the fragrant herbal elixir out over your body.

HELPFUL HINTS

Most health food stores will have a muslin bag available in the tea, herbal, or body care section. You can also use a clean sock or nylon, or tie the herbal mix in a piece of cheesecloth or other soft natural fabric.

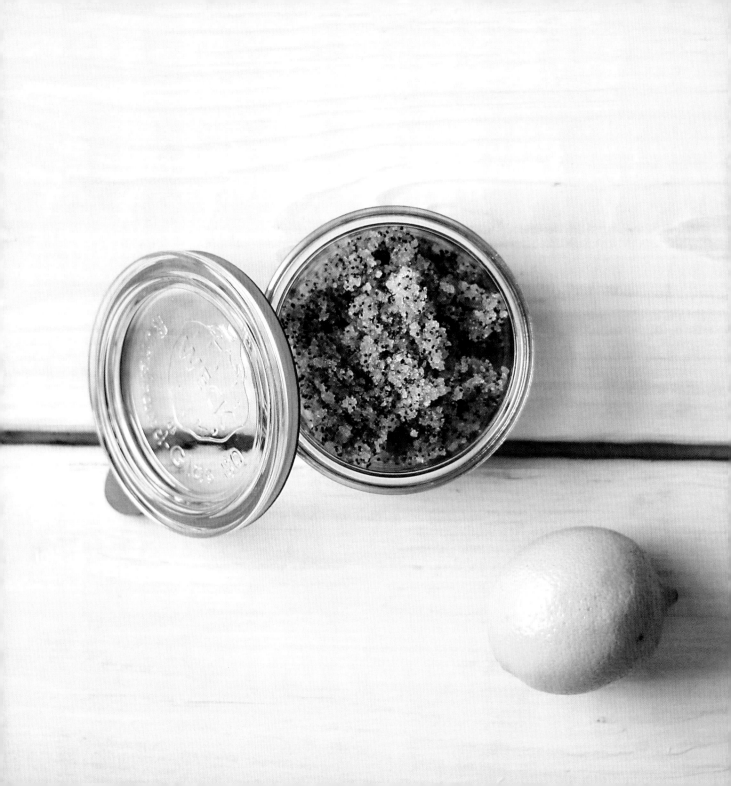

Lemon Poppy Seed SCRUB

The Roman goddess of youth was symbolized by the lemon, which grows wild in the sun-soaked Mediterranean. This recipe is naturally high in vitamin C, which combats premature aging, lightens brown spots, helps balance oil production, and fights acne. Tart and tangy lemons, spicy cardamom, and poppy seeds come together in this sweet and citrusy wonderscrub for your body-beautiful skin care routine.

YIELDS: *about 8 ounces*

2 tablespoons poppy seeds

½ cup granulated sugar

Dash of ground cardamom

Zest of ½ lemon

¼ cup grapeseed oil

1 teaspoon fresh lemon juice

What you will need: mixing bowl, measuring cups, fork, jars and lids to fit 8 ounces of scrub

1 To Make: Place the poppy seeds, sugar, cardamom, and lemon zest in a medium-size mixing bowl. Add the oil and mix together with a fork until you have a uniform consistency. Lastly, add the lemon juice and stir well to blend.

2 To Store: To preserve the freshness of this natural scrub, keep water out of it. Store this scrub in a sealed container in the refrigerator and use up within a week.

3 To Use: Use in place of a soap or body wash in your shower or bath. Apply to damp skin in small, upward motions. Massage the scrub in small circular motions, starting with the legs and arms, making your way up to the torso, ending at your heart. Rinse well.

SKIN CARE SECRETS

When applying a body scrub, use small circular motions and light pressure. Avoid any open wounds, especially with a salt scrub, and use caution as the shower floor may become slippery.

Invigorating GINGER CITRUS BODY WASH

Ginger and citrus make a divine scent combination that is also great for your mind, body, and spirit. Warming, soothing, and revitalizing to the senses, this body wash is great for invigorating your skin cells, increasing circulation, detoxification, and promoting a more radiant skin tone.

YIELDS: *9 ounces*

¼ cup finely chopped fresh ginger

½ cup sweet almond oil

2 tablespoons honey

10 drops lime essential oil

8 drops lemon essential oil

12 drops pink grapefruit essential oil

½ cup unscented liquid Castile soap

What you will need: cutting board, knife, double boiler, strainer, mixing bowl, wire whisk, funnel, measuring cups, 8–9-ounce bottle and cap

1 **To Make:** Start the double boiler on medium heat. Once it reaches a boil, reduce heat to simmer. Place the chopped ginger and sweet almond oil in the top of the double boiler and cover. Simmer for 30–45 minutes, stirring occasionally. To preserve the beneficial botanicals, do not overheat and check back every 20 minutes to make sure there's enough water in the double boiler. Remove from heat; take the top pan off the double boiler. Strain the ginger from the oil into the mixing bowl, using the rubber spatula to get the remainder out of the pan. Add the honey and whisk together for a minute. Add the essential oils and whisk to blend. Next, add the Castile soap, stirring gently with the whisk to create a uniform liquid. Do not overwhisk, as this activates the soap bubbles. Use the funnel to carefully pour into your bottle and cap tightly.

2 **To Store:** Store in bottle. Label with contents and date and use within a year.

3 **To Use:** Use as body wash in your shower or bath. Apply to damp skin in small, upward motions. Rinse well.

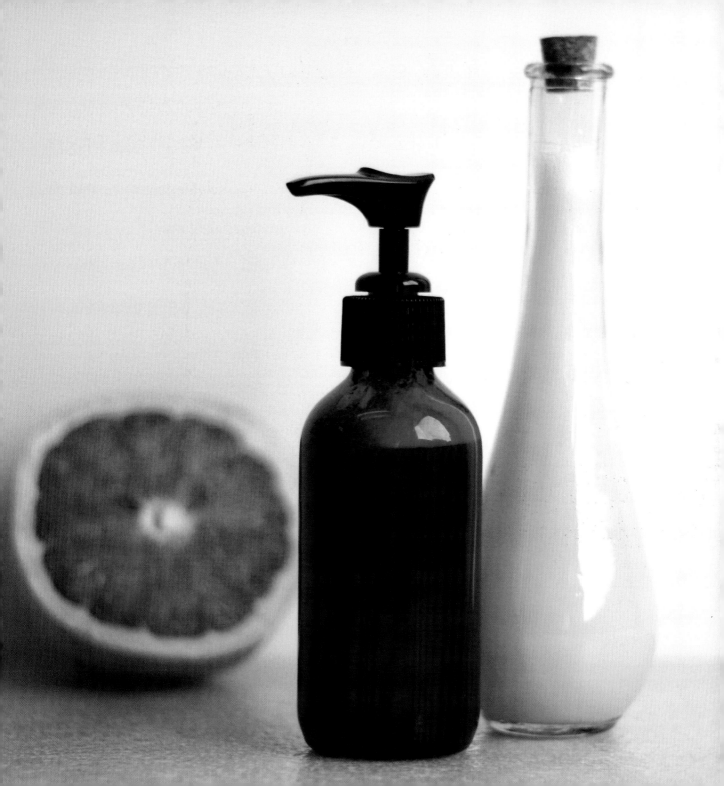

Shea Butter
BODY WASH

This formula is super moisturizing, creamy, and very easy to make! Add scent and therapeutic skin care benefits by substituting one of the infused oils from Chapter 7 for the sweet almond oil and/or add your favorite essential oil blend from Appendix A. You could also start with a scented Castile soap and have fun with creative scent layering to make a one-of-a-kind scent.

YIELDS: *16 ounces*

½ cup shea butter

1 cup unscented liquid Castile soap

½ cup sweet almond oil

2 x essential oil blend, optional
  (see Appendix A)

What you will need: double boiler, funnel, measuring cups, 16-ounce bottle and cap

1 **To Make:** Start the double boiler on medium heat. Once it reaches a boil, reduce heat to simmer. Place the shea butter in the top of the double boiler and cover. Simmer until melted, stirring occasionally. To preserve the beneficial botanicals, do not overheat. Remove from heat and take the top pan off the double boiler and wipe dry with a towel. Using a funnel, carefully pour the Castile soap and sweet almond oil into the bottle and add the essential oils. Pour the melted shea butter into the bottle; use a rubber spatula to get the remainder out of the pan. Cap tightly and gently shake for a few minutes to blend the ingredients.

2 **To Store:** Store in bottle, away from direct sunlight. Label with contents and date and use within a year.

3 **To Use:** Use as body wash in your shower or bath. Apply to damp skin in small, upward motions. Rinse well.

Honey Coconut
BODY WASH

Gorgeous moisture from the coconut oil, invigorating antibacterial properties of the honey, and a tangy touch of citrus make this body wash unique. You will have a home spa day with every shower when you use this luxurious, honey-sweet, coconutty, sunshine-scented moisturizing body wash.

YIELDS: *16 ounces*

½ cup extra-virgin coconut oil

½ cup raw honey

20 drops sweet orange essential oil

10 drops lemon essential oil

6 drops chamomile essential oil

1 cup unscented liquid Castile soap

What you will need: double boiler, mixing bowl, wire whisk, funnel, measuring cups, 16-ounce bottle and cap

1 To Make: Start the double boiler on medium heat. Once it reaches a boil, reduce heat to simmer. Place the coconut oil in the top of the double boiler and cover. Simmer until it's melted, stirring occasionally. To preserve the beneficial botanicals, do not overheat. Remove from heat; take the top pan off the double boiler and wipe it dry with a towel. Put the honey into the mixing bowl and add the coconut oil, using the rubber spatula to get the remainder out of the pan. Whisk the ingredients together for a minute. Add the essential oils and whisk to blend. Next, add the Castile soap, stirring gently with the whisk to create a uniform liquid. Do not overwhisk, as this activates the soap bubbles. Use the funnel to carefully pour into your bottle and cap tightly.

2 To Store: Store in bottle. Label with contents and date and use within a year.

3 To Use: Use as body wash in your shower or bath. Apply to damp skin in small, upward motions. Rinse well.

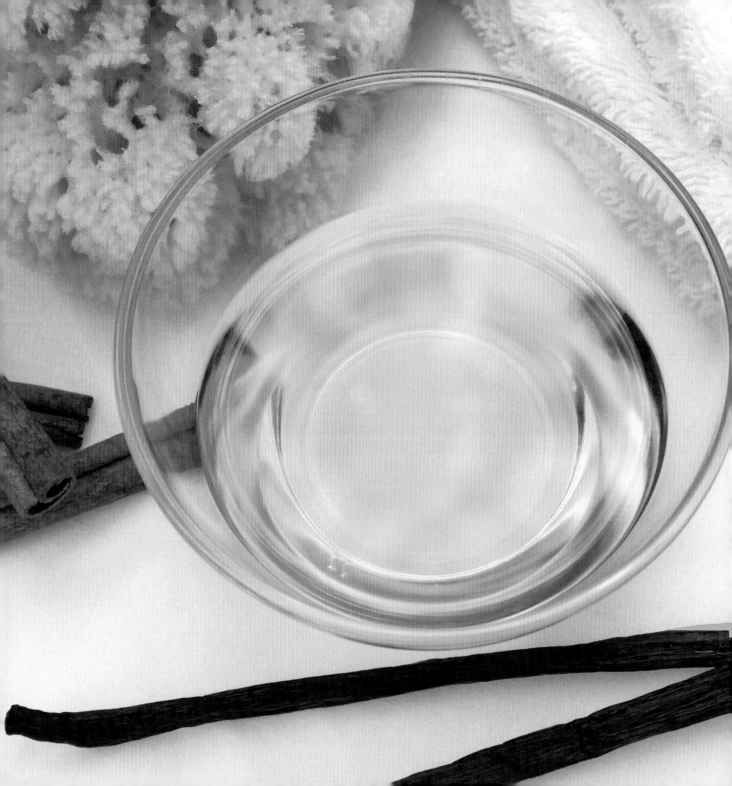

CHAPTER 5

BODY BUTTERS AND OILS

Let's face it: your skin is quite miraculous! It is the largest organ of your body and it is constantly renewing itself. It shields you from the weather and from environmental hazards. It's the outer shell that holds us all together. On a good day it's your soft pretty covering. And on a bad day it's itchy, dry, irritated, and inflamed.

One of the best things you can do for your skin is to help it stay moisturized. The nutrient-rich botanical moisturizers found in this chapter are formulated to create a protective, regenerative barrier that softens dry or cracked skin, restoring natural elasticity. My all-time favorite skin care ingredients come straight from nature's pharmacy and include shea butter, jojoba oil, grapeseed oil, and, of course, essential oils. You'll find these amazing natural emollients and more in these easy-to-make, ultra-lush recipes like the Coco-Spice Body Butter, Warm Cinnamon Massage Oil, and Cuticle Saver Treatment found in this chapter. So get ready to slather yourself in moisturizing goodness. Your skin will thank you!

BODY BUTTER
Bars

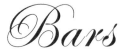

These Body Butter Bars—also known as solid lotion or lotion bars—are easy and fun to make. They work like typical body butters, but in a bar form. They melt with the heat of your skin, so all you need to do is rub one over dry skin like you would a bar of soap; it leaves behind a rich and lovely moisturizing layer on your skin. Unlike lotion, these bars don't have a water element, so they don't need a chemical preservative. They're great as a daily moisturizer and for massage. Leave them unscented and they work wonders for combating stretch marks on pregnant bellies. These Body Butter Bars can be packaged up very nicely as gifts or party favors.

YIELDS: *7 ounces*

2 tablespoons grated beeswax

¼ cup shea butter

¼ cup coconut oil (virgin or unscented)

¼ cup sweet almond oil

4 vitamin E capsules

Essential oil blend (see Appendix A)

What you will need: double boiler, measuring cups, rubber spatula, push-up tubes

❶ **To Make:** Start the double boiler on medium heat. Once it reaches a boil, reduce heat to simmer. Place the beeswax, shea butter, and coconut oil in the top of the double boiler and cover. Simmer until melted, stirring occasionally. To preserve the beneficial botanicals, do not overheat. Remove from heat, take the top pan off the double boiler, and cool 5–10 minutes. Add the sweet almond oil. Pierce the vitamin E capsules and squeeze the liquid out into the melted oil, discarding the gel caps. Add the essential oil blend and stir well, scraping any of the hardened cooled mixture off the sides and back into the melted oils. If the mixture hardens too much before you can pour it, gently melt it again in the double boiler. Pour into the lotion tubes and let stand undisturbed for 4 hours or overnight before use.

2 **To Store:** Label and use within 1 year. Store out of direct sunlight.

3 **To Use:** Solid lotion bars will melt on contact with your warm skin, allowing you to apply just the right amount of moisturizer, exactly where you need it. Rub it into your cuticles and the cracks in your hands, elbows, and feet. Apply to dry skin as needed.

HELPFUL HINTS

You can make this recipe into bars (like soap) instead of the push-up tubes. Follow the directions given. Pour the melted butter into an ice cube tray, silicone mold, or a loaf pan lined with wax paper. Let stand at least 4 hours before moving. The hardened bars should easily pop out of the molds. If not, place in the freezer for 10 minutes, then carefully run hot water on the backside of the mold. Quickly dry it off with a towel and twist the mold to remove. If you chose a loaf pan, use a warm knife to cut the bars at least 1" thick. Store these lotion bars in metal tins, wrapped in foil, or in a glass jar.

Healing
COMFREY SALVE

Comfrey has been used for centuries to accelerate healing for all manner of skin conditions. This recipe incorporates green tea and chamomile for amplified anti-inflammatory, soothing, and regenerative benefits. You can use this Healing Comfrey Salve as a hand and body butter or as an intensive healing salve.

YIELDS: *8 ounces*

¼ cup beeswax

½ cup Fresh Comfrey Oil (see Chapter 7)

¼ cup Green Tea–Infused Oil (see Chapter 7)

2 vitamin E capsules

12 drops chamomile essential oil

What you will need: double boiler, measuring cups, rubber spatula, jars with lids to hold 8 ounces of balm

1 **To Make:** Start the double boiler on medium heat. Once it reaches a boil reduce heat to simmer. Place the beeswax in the top of the double boiler and cover. Simmer until melted, stirring occasionally. To preserve the beneficial nutrients, do not overheat. Remove from heat, take the top pan off the double boiler, and cool 5–10 minutes. Add the Fresh Comfrey Oil and Green Tea–Infused Oil to the melted beeswax and stir. Pierce the vitamin E capsules and squeeze the liquid out into the melted oil, discarding the gel caps. Add the essential oil and stir well, scraping any of the hardened cooled mixture off the sides and back into the melted oils. If the mixture hardens too much before you can pour it, gently melt it again in the double boiler. Pour into your jars and let stand undisturbed for 4 hours or overnight before use.

2 **To Store:** Label and store in a cool dry place away from direct sunlight. Use within a year.

3 **To Use:** Simply remove a small amount from the jar and melt between your fingertips, then spread it into your cuticles and the cracks in your hands, elbows, and feet. Take advantage of the natural healing properties and apply to bruises, superficial burns, diaper rash, blisters, cuts, and more. Do not use on open wounds. Reapply often for best results.

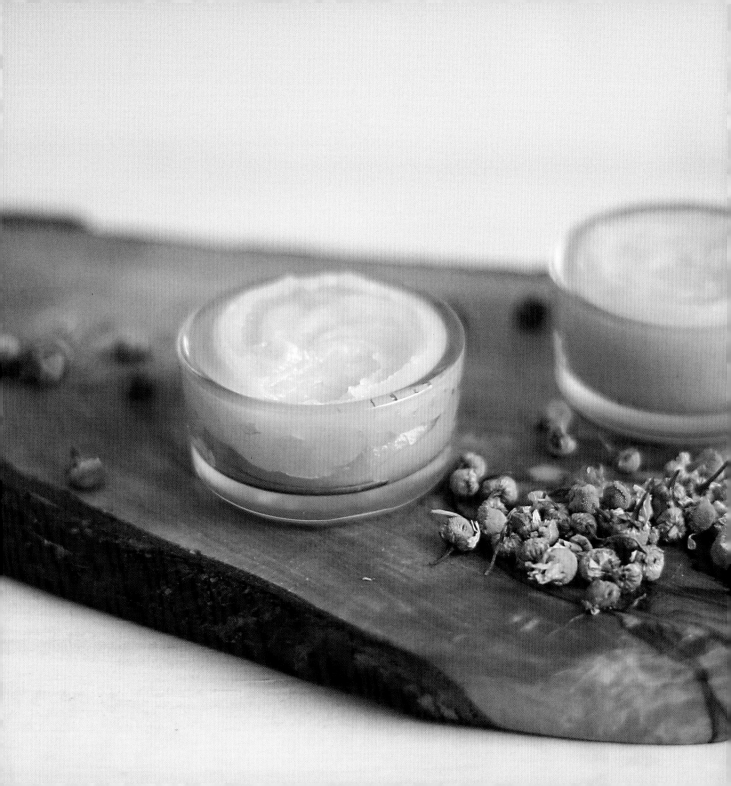

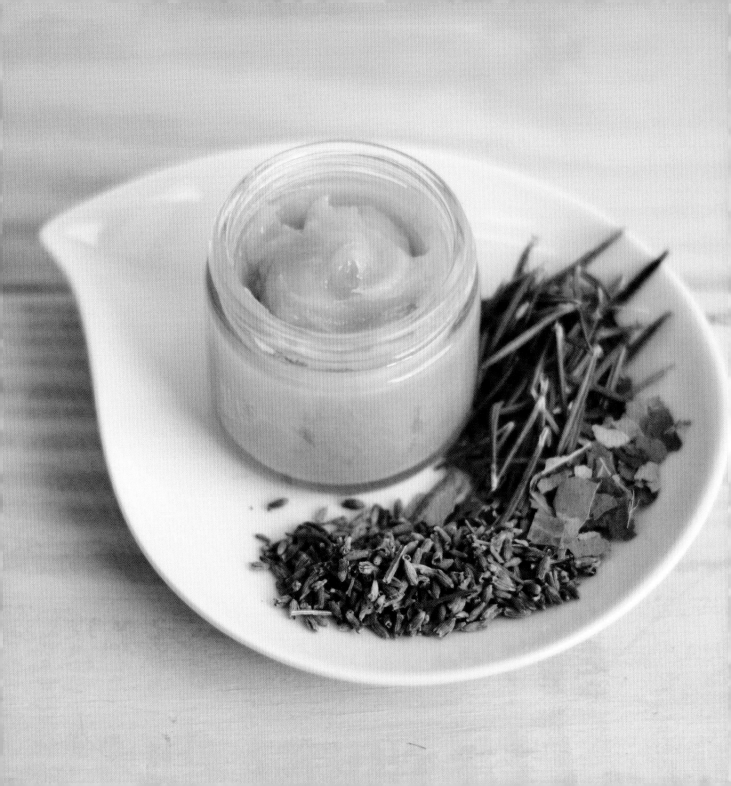

Gardener's
HERBAL BALM

This silky, buttery balm with a sweet herbal scent works to soothe, hydrate, and protect your work-weary hands. The skin on your hands is hard to keep moist because it is thin and has relatively few oil glands. It is beneficial to apply this herbal balm right after gardening, knitting, dishwashing, rock climbing, or playing sports. It's lovely just to rub some into your hands while watching TV or talking on the phone. This soothing herbal balm is so light, you will want to use it all over!

YIELDS: *8 ounces*

¼ cup grated beeswax

¼ cup coconut oil (unscented)

¼ cup Fresh Comfrey Oil (see Chapter 7)

¼ cup Fresh Herbal Oil (see Chapter 7)

2 vitamin E capsules

20 drops eucalyptus essential oil

20 drops lavender essential oil

What you will need: double boiler, measuring cups, rubber spatula, jars to hold 8 ounces of balm

❶ **To Make:** Start the double boiler on medium heat. Once it reaches a boil, reduce heat to simmer. Place the beeswax and coconut oil in the top of the double boiler and cover. Simmer until melted, stirring occasionally. To preserve the beneficial nutrients, do not overheat. Remove from heat, take the top pan off the double boiler, and cool 5–10 minutes. Add the Fresh Comfrey Oil and Fresh Herbal Oil to the pot and stir. Pierce the vitamin E capsules and squeeze the liquid out into the melted oil, discarding the gel caps. Add the essential oils and stir well, scraping any of the hardened cooled mixture off the sides and back into the melted oils. If the mixture hardens too much before you can pour it, gently melt it again in the double boiler. Pour into your jars and let stand undisturbed for 4 hours or overnight before use.

❷ **To Store:** Label jars and store in a cool dry place away from direct sunlight. Use within a year.

❸ **To Use:** Remove a small amount from the jar and melt between your fingertips, then spread it into your cuticles and the cracks in your hands, elbows, and feet.

Whipped SHEA BODY BUTTER

This recipe makes a light and fluffy shea buttery moisturizer that you can use from head to toe. It works to keep beneficial moisture locked in while letting your skin breathe. Customize this recipe by adding your favorite essential oil blend or using an infused oil from Chapter 7 instead of the olive oil.

YIELDS: *10 ounces by weight*

The volume will vary depending on how much air you are able to whip into the final product. Plan for this and have enough jars to hold 14 ounces by volume.

⅔ cup shea butter

¼ cup coconut oil

¼ cup olive oil, or favorite infused oil from Chapter 7

4 vitamin E capsules

Essential oil blend, optional (see Appendix A)

What you will need: measuring cups, double boiler, mixing bowl, electric mixer, rubber spatula, jars with lids to hold 10–14 ounces of butter

❶ To Make: Start the double boiler on medium heat. Once it reaches a boil, reduce heat to simmer. Place the shea butter in the top of the double boiler and cover. Simmer until almost all the way melted, stirring occasionally. To preserve the beneficial nutrients, do not overheat. Remove from heat, take the top pan off the double boiler, and wipe with a towel so no water drips into your melted butter. Pour into the mixing bowl and use the rubber spatula to get all of the melted shea out of the pan. Add the coconut and olive oils and allow to cool 10–15 minutes. Stir the oils, scraping the hardening butter off the sides of the bowl. If you have a whisk attachment to your electric mixer, use it. Otherwise, the regular beaters will work fine. Beat on medium for 5 minutes. Scrape the sides of the bowl with the rubber spatula. Pierce the vitamin E capsules and squeeze the liquid out into the melted oil, discarding the gel caps. Add the essential oils, if desired, and stir well. If the mixture is still quite liquid, place in the freezer for 5 minutes. Mix for another 5 minutes. Repeat the 5 minutes in the freezer, 5 minutes mixing process until you have a fluffy, smooth, buttery texture. Spoon into your jars and let stand undisturbed for an hour.

❷ To Store: Label and store in a cool dry place away from direct sunlight. This butter will melt if left in the sun. It will still be useable, but the nice fluffy quality from the whipping will be gone. It will revert to a solid butter balm consistency. Use within a year.

❸ To Use: Remove a small amount from the jar and melt between your fingertips and spread onto dry skin.

Lovely BODY BUTTER

Hydrating, nourishing, and replenishing, this vegan body butter quenches dry skin, leaving you soft and glowing. This combination of natural butters forms a protective, regenerative moisturizer that is beneficial for all skin types.

YIELDS: *8 ounces*

¾ cup unscented cocoa butter

1 tablespoon coconut oil

2 tablespoons sweet almond oil

4 vitamin E capsules

30–40 drops of essential oils, optional (see sidebar, page 98)

What you will need: measuring cups, double boiler, rubber spatula, jars to hold 8 ounces of balm, plastic wrap

① **To Make:** Start the double boiler on medium heat. Once it reaches a boil, reduce heat to simmer. Place the cocoa butter in the top of the double boiler and cover. Simmer until it is melted, stirring occasionally. To preserve the beneficial nutrients, do not overheat. Remove from heat, take the top pan off the double boiler, and dry off with a towel so no water drips into your melted butter. Add the coconut oil and stir until it is melted. Add the sweet almond oil and stir. Let stand for 10 minutes, or until the oils have cooled to the touch but are not yet forming a hard layer around the edges of the pan. Pierce the vitamin E capsules and squeeze the liquid out into the melted oil, discarding the gel caps. Add the essential oils if desired and stir well, scraping any of the hardened cooled mixture off the sides and back into the melted oils. Pour into jars, cover with plastic wrap, and let stand undisturbed for 4 hours or overnight.

② **To Store:** Put the jar lids on tightly and label with contents and expiration date of 1 year. Store in a cool dry place away from direct sunlight.

③ **To Use:** Remove a small amount from the jar and melt between your fingertips and spread onto dry skin.

(continued on the following page)

SKIN CARE SECRETS

Note that this formula is unscented. There are several fun ways to incorporate scent into this formula: Substitute the sweet almond oil for an infused oil from Chapter 7; use an essential oil blend from Appendix A; use scented versus unscented cocoa butter or coconut oil. You can get creative and layer an essential oil blend with an infused oil, such as the Sunny Day Blend with the Lavender-Infused Oil, or choose extra-virgin coconut oil with the Hippie Love Blend, etc. Whatever you decide to do, have fun, get creative, and mix it up!

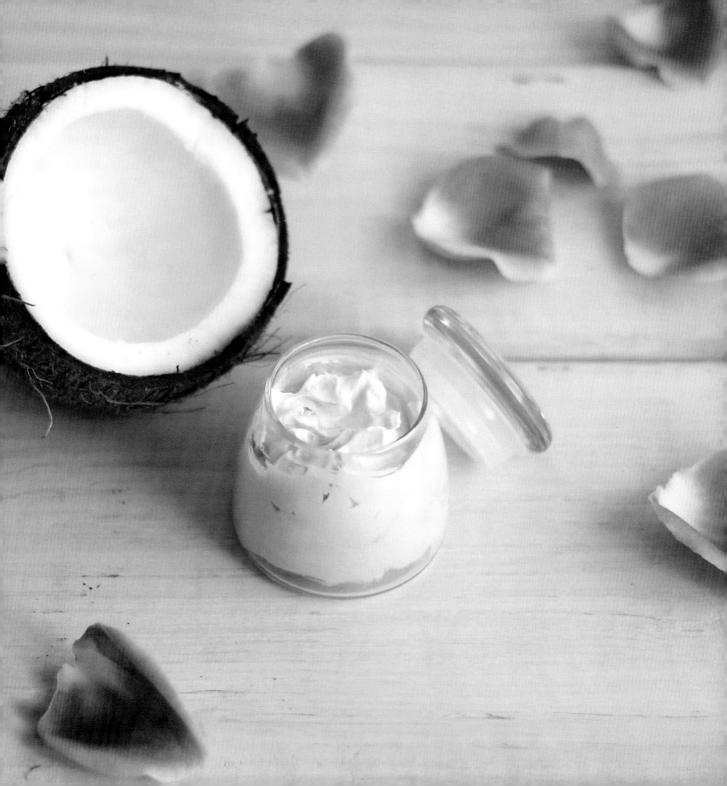

Coco-Spice
BODY BUTTER

This Coco-Spice Body Butter is gorgeously warm and spicy with hints of chocolate and coconut. This is homemade luxury at its best!

YIELDS: *about 10 ounces*

2 teaspoons grated beeswax

½ cup cocoa butter

2 tablespoons extra-virgin coconut oil

½ cup Chai Spice–Infused Oil (see Chapter 7)

12 drops patchouli essential oil

20 drops sweet orange essential oil

4 vitamin E capsules

What you will need: measuring cups, double boiler, rubber spatula, jars to hold 10 ounces of balm

1 **To Make:** Start the double boiler on medium heat. Once it reaches a boil, reduce heat to simmer. Place the beeswax and cocoa butter in the top of the double boiler and cover. Simmer until it is melted, stirring occasionally. To preserve the beneficial nutrients, do not overheat. Remove from heat, take the top pan off the double boiler, and dry with a towel so no water drips into your melted butter. Add the coconut oil and stir until it is melted. Add the Chai Spice–Infused Oil and stir. Let stand for 10 minutes, or until the oils have cooled to the touch but are not yet forming a hard layer around the edges of the pan. At this point stir in the essential oils. Pierce the vitamin E capsules and squeeze the liquid out into the melted oil, discarding the gel caps. Stir well, scraping any of the hardened cooled mixture off the sides and back into the melted oils. Pour into your jars, cover with plastic wrap, and let stand undisturbed for 4 hours or overnight.

2 **To Store:** Put the jar lids on tightly and label with contents and date. Store in a cool dry place away from direct sunlight and use within a year.

3 **To Use:** Remove a small amount from the jar and melt between your fingertips and spread onto dry skin.

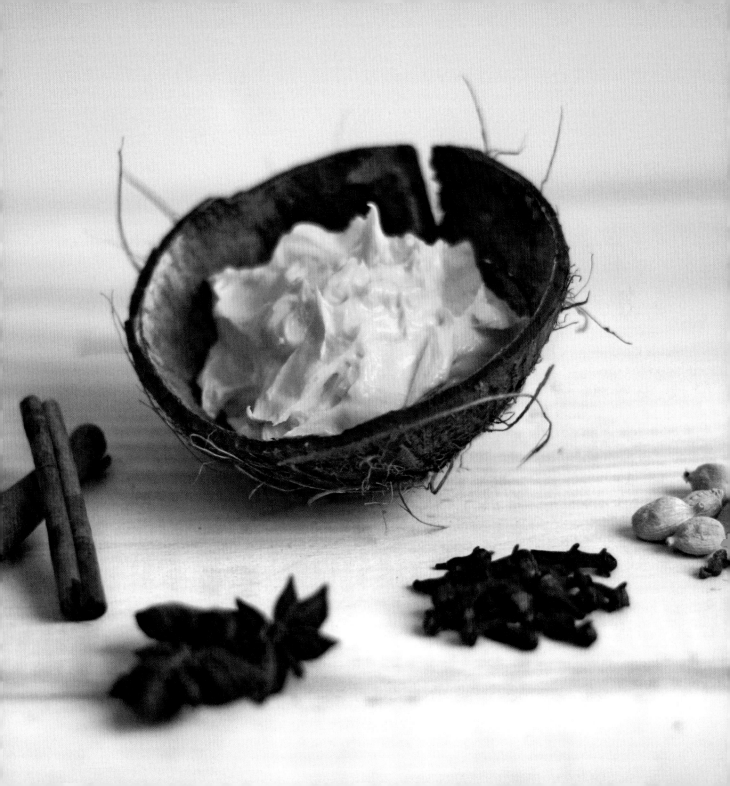

Luxurious BODY OIL

Nourishing, conditioning, and moisturizing, body oils are a luxurious alternative to lotions. Lotion contains up to 80 percent water that evaporates off of your skin with little therapeutic value. However, a properly formulated body oil is pure, concentrated moisture that is rich in botanical nutrients.

YIELDS: *8 ounces*

¼ cup Green Tea–Infused Oil (see Chapter 7)

½ cup jojoba oil

¼ cup sweet almond oil

4 vitamin E capsules

Essential oil blend, optional

What you will need: measuring cups, funnel, dark-colored 8-ounce bottle with cap (pump top optional)

1 **To Make:** Place the funnel over your bottle and add the oils. Pierce the vitamin E capsules and squeeze the liquid out into the bottle, discarding the gel caps. Add the essential oils, if desired. Place the cap on tightly, and shake to blend.

2 **To Store:** Label with contents and expiration date. Will keep for up to a year.

3 **To Use:** Apply to dry skin as needed.

HELPFUL HINTS

Pure, undiluted jojoba oil is generally considered to have a long shelf life of 2 or more years if stored out of direct sunlight. It is expensive, but if you desire a longer shelf life for any of the products that use a liquid oil in this book, you can substitute jojoba oil. Substituting jojoba oil will change the consistency and nutrient content of the final product and prolong freshness, but the shelf life will be dependent on the sum total of the ingredients in the recipe.

Sore Muscle
MASSAGE OIL

This intensive blend of botanicals is perfect for soothing and relaxing your sore, tired muscles. The carrot seed oil is particularly helpful for reducing accumulation of toxins in muscles and joints and lessening inflammation to benefit arthritis and rheumatism relief. Massage this Sore Muscle Massage Oil onto your neck and shoulders to relieve stress or rub into sore muscles after a workout for a natural herbal relief.

YIELDS: *8 ounces*

⅓ cup extra-virgin olive oil

⅓ cup herbal-infused oil (see Chapter 7) or jojoba oil

⅓ cup sweet almond oil

16 drops carrot seed essential oil

8 drops chamomile essential oil

12 drops lavender essential oil

4 vitamin E capsules

What you will need: funnel, dark-colored 8-ounce bottle with cap (pump top optional)

❶ **To Make:** Place the funnel over your blending container and add the oils. Pierce the vitamin E capsules and squeeze the liquid out into the container, discarding the gel caps. Add the essential oils and shake to blend.

❷ **To Store:** Label with contents and expiration date. Will keep for up to a year. Store out of direct sunlight.

❸ **To Use:** Apply to sore muscles and joints as needed.

HELPFUL HINTS

To help prolong the freshness of your natural creations and preserve the oils, you want your storage bottle to have as little air space as possible. Choose a dark container to help slow the oxidation process of the active botanical oils, which will prolong the product's shelf life and maintain the integrity of the active botanical ingredients.

Warm Cinnamon
MASSAGE OIL

You will love the silky texture of this massage oil, especially on a cold night, as it brings a deep warming sensation to your skin, muscles, and joints. The cozy cinnamon scent makes this great massage oil a perfect comfort for the colder weather months. The warming spices work to soothe sore, aching muscles after exercise or a long day's work.

YIELDS: *8 ounces*

2 cinnamon sticks

5 whole cloves

1 teaspoon fresh chopped ginger

¼ cup jojoba oil

¼ cup olive oil

¼ cup sweet almond oil

¼ cup coconut oil

4 vitamin E capsules

16 drops patchouli essential oil

What you will need: double boiler, measuring cups, mesh strainer, rubber spatula, 8-ounce Mason jar or bottle (pump top optional), funnel

❶ **To Make:** Start the double boiler on medium heat. Once it reaches a boil, reduce heat to simmer. Break up the cinnamon sticks and place in the top of the double boiler along with the cloves and ginger. Cover the spices with the jojoba, olive, almond, and coconut oils and cover. Simmer on low heat for at least an hour, stirring occasionally. To preserve the beneficial botanicals, do not overheat. Remove from heat, take the top pan off the double boiler, and let cool. Strain the spices from the oil and use the funnel to pour the oil into an 8-ounce Mason jar or bottle. Pierce the vitamin E capsules and squeeze the liquid out into the bottle, discarding the gel caps. Add the essential oil, cap tightly, and shake to blend.

❷ **To Store:** Label with contents and expiration date. Will keep for up to a year. Store away from heat and out of direct sunlight.

❸ **To Use:** Use as an all-over massage oil. You may also use this as a body oil by applying to dry skin as desired.

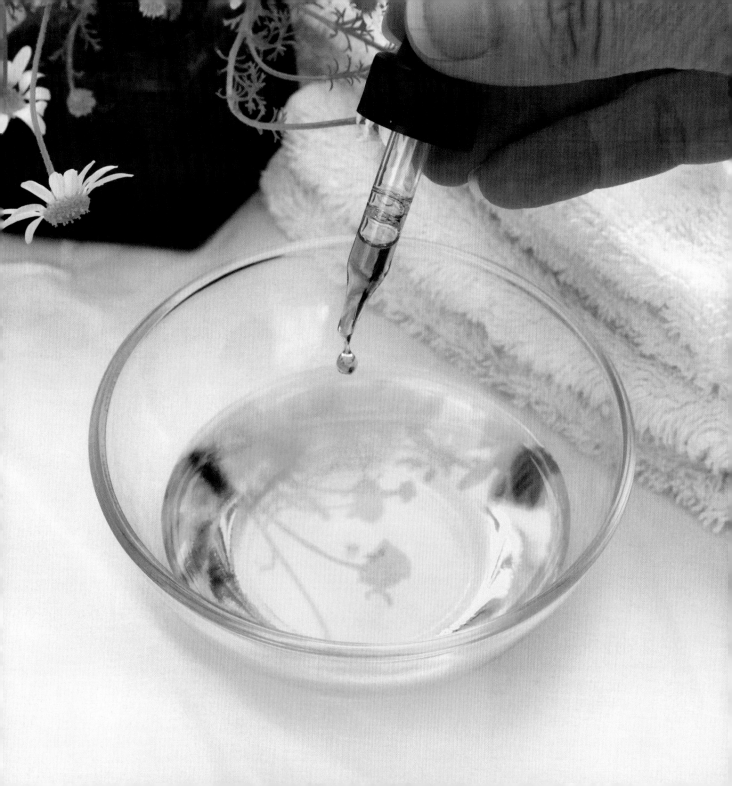

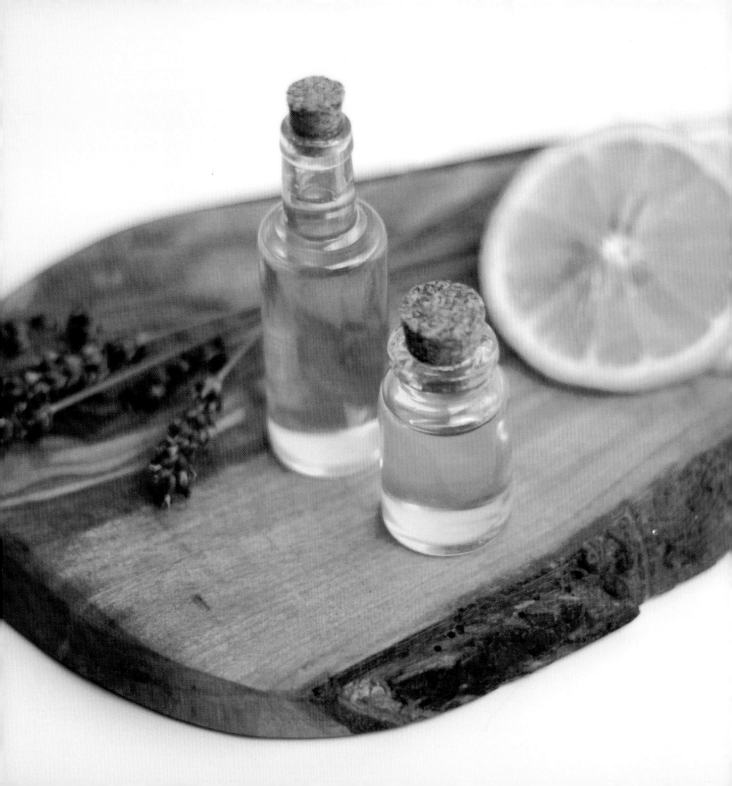

CUTICLE SAVER
Treatment

If you do housework, garden, bite your nails, knit, cook, or work in any profession in which
you need to wash your hands constantly, you probably know what unhappy cuticles feel like.
Soothe, condition, and repair them with this luxurious botanical treatment serum.

YIELDS: *1 ounce*

2 teaspoons extra-virgin olive oil

2 teaspoons herbal-infused oil (see
Chapter 7) or jojoba oil

1 teaspoon grapeseed oil, unscented

16 drops tea tree essential oil

12 drops lemon essential oil

12 drops lavender essential oil

1 vitamin E capsule

What you will need: dark-
colored 1-ounce bottle with a
dropper top, small funnel

❶ **To Make:** Place the funnel over your bottle and add the oils. Pierce the
vitamin E capsule and squeeze it out into the bottle, discarding the gel
cap. Add the essential oils and shake to blend.

❷ **To Store:** Label with contents and expiration date of 6 months. Store
out of direct sunlight.

❸ **To Use:** Use daily for improved nail and cuticle health. Apply a few
drops before bedtime, massaging the serum into your fingernails, the
surrounding cuticle skin, and your hands. Using this serum before bed
allows the serum to work its magic throughout the night while you
are sleeping. For a deeply healing, moisturizing treatment, massage a
generous amount of the Cuticle Saver Treatment into the cuticles and
fingernails. Leave on for 10–30 minutes, allowing the serum to work
its botanical magic. This blend absorbs very quickly, so there probably
won't be any excess, but if there is, wipe off with a clean dry cloth. This
deep treatment works best on unpolished fingernails.

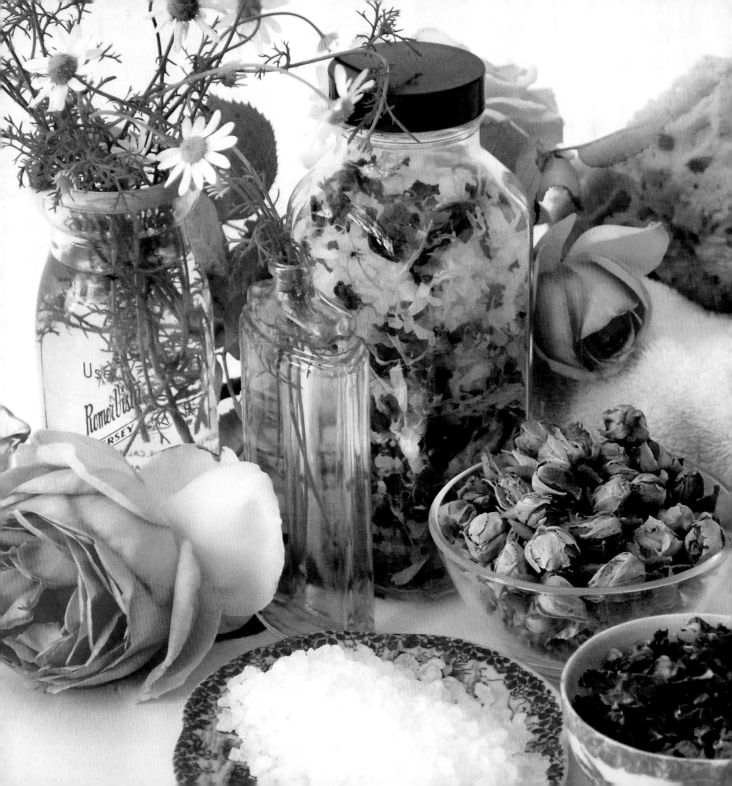

CHAPTER 6

BATHS

The art of the bath is a true luxury. The pace of our modern life demands that we be quick about most everything, but it sure is worthwhile to carve out the time for a bath. Schedule at least an hour and dedicate this time to incorporating at least a couple of beauty treatments into your bath time. Set a lovely scene for yourself as your tub fills. Turn off the phone, light some candles, and let the luxury begin! If your home doesn't have a bathtub, don't despair! Invest in a washtub and give yourself a foot bath. Surprisingly, soaking your feet is one of the best ways to absorb essential oils and beneficial vitamins and minerals into your bloodstream. Not to mention how good it feels to soak your tired feet in a soothing bath after a long day's work.

Choose a bath treatment to suit your mood or specific needs. If you're feeling under the weather, choose the Angel Soak for Cold and Flu and rub some herbal-infused oil (Chapter 7) on your chest and use it as a hand treatment. If you are in a fun, playful mood, toss a couple of Bath Fizzies into your tub and give yourself a colorful facial using the Aztec Honey and Wine Mask (Chapter 3). If your skin is feeling dry and itchy, opt for a luxurious moisturizing Bath Melt and melt those cares away. With so many fabulous options at your fingertips, a fantastic bath time spa experience is definitely in your future!

Coconut, Lime, and Rose Petals BATH

This luxurious bath is made from coconut milk, lime slices, and heaps of fresh rose petals for a tropically inspired bath time escape to another world. With soothing, replenishing, anti-inflammatory properties, this bath increases circulation and encourages detoxification while moisturizing the skin. Bathing in lime, roses, and coconut is particularly beneficial for dry skin conditions, including sunburn and eczema. These aromatic and strikingly beautiful fresh ingredients delight your senses while pampering, nourishing, and conditioning for petal-soft skin.

YIELDS: *1 bath*

½ cup fresh rose petals

1 lime

1 cup coconut milk

What you will need: knife, cutting board

1. **To Make:** Remove the petals from the roses directly after cutting from the plant to preserve the highest nutrient value and reserve. Slice the lime into rounds. Draw a bath. When the tub is almost full, add all ingredients to the water and swish around.

2. **To Store:** Plan to make this bath recipe fresh for each use.

3. **To Use:** Soak for at least 20 minutes, or longer to enjoy maximum therapeutic benefits of the active botanical ingredients. When you are finished soaking, rinse off in the shower to remove the sweat and toxins you released as you bathed. After a bath is also the perfect time to use a body scrub, as your skin is softened and easily exfoliated. The Citrus Blast Body Scrub (Chapter 4) is ideal. Follow with moisturizer if desired.

HELPFUL HINTS

Choose robustly blooming roses to pluck the petals from for this recipe. Pick them from your garden midmorning, after the dew has dried but before they wilt with the heat of the day.

Mermaid BATH

Mystical mermaids have beautifully glowing skin because they are constantly replenishing themselves by bathing in the sea. This Mermaid Bath uses seaweed full of rich vitamins, minerals, trace elements, and amino acids to extract toxins from your body and relax your muscles. The lavender and spearmint bring a fresh herbal scent to this mellow, detoxifying, and replenishing bath that is beneficial for all skin types.

YIELDS: *1 pint*

1½ cups solar-dried sea salt

40 drops pink grapefruit essential oil

¼ cup dried lavender buds

⅛ cup dried spearmint

2 teaspoons dried bladderwrack

1 tablespoon dried kelp

What you will need: mixing bowl, spoon, pint jar with lid, cloth bag or cheesecloth, and string to make a sachet

1 **To Make:** Place the salts in the bowl. Stir in the pink grapefruit essential oil in intervals. Add a little, stir, add a little more, stir, until you have added all 40 drops and mixed them into the salt. Add the lavender, spearmint, and seaweeds. Stir until you have a uniform blend.

2 **To Store:** Store in a sealed jar labeled with contents and expiration date of 6 months.

3 **To Use:** Draw a bath. Make a sachet loosely filled with the salt mixture and toss into the tub. When the tub is full, get in and soak for at least 20 minutes, or longer to enjoy maximum therapeutic benefits of the active botanical ingredients. Use the sachet as a wash bag or compress. Gently squeeze the liquid from the sachet over your skin and relax while your mind, body, and spirit are replenished. When you are finished soaking, rinse off in the shower to remove the sweat and toxins you released as you bathed. After a bath is also the perfect time to use the Herb Garden Body Scrub (see Chapter 4), as your skin is softened and easily exfoliated. If you do not use a body scrub, use your favorite moisturizer to seal in the nutrients and complete the home spa experience.

Sunshine C BATH

This skin-softening combination of oranges and hibiscus is beneficial for all skin types, including oily, acne-prone, maturing, and sun-damaged. The high levels of antioxidants and vitamin C in this formula stimulate cellular renewal, promote collagen formation, and fight against premature aging. As the hibiscus infuses into the bath water, your tub will become the most beautiful vitamin C–infused sunset of pinkish purple and orange water. Enjoy!

YIELDS: *1 bath*

1 cup solar-dried sea salt

1 tablespoon dried hibiscus flowers

1 small orange

1 teaspoon carrier oil of choice, optional

Fresh or dried rose petals, optional

What you will need: knife, cutting board, cloth bag, tea ball or cheesecloth and string

❶ **To Make:** Draw a bath. Put the sea salt into the tub. Place the hibiscus into the cloth bag and toss into the tub. Slice the orange into rounds. Add the carrier oil if you desire the added moisture. When the tub is full, add the oranges and rose petals, if desired, to the water and swish around.

❷ **To Store:** Plan to make this fresh for each use.

❸ **To Use:** Get in the tub and soak for at least 20 minutes, or longer to enjoy maximum therapeutic benefits of the active botanical ingredients. When you are finished soaking, rinse off in the shower to remove the sweat and toxins you released as you bathed. After a bath is also the perfect time to use a body scrub, as your skin is softened and easily exfoliated. The Valencia Coffee Scrub from Chapter 4 is ideal. Follow with moisturizer if desired.

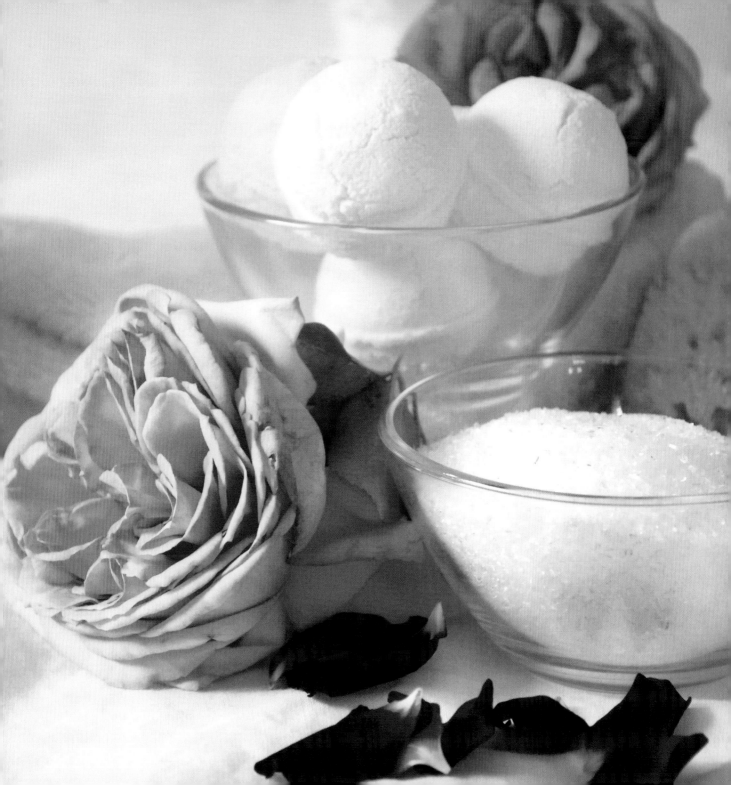

Bath MELTS

Bath Melts are a super-moisturizing bath treat guaranteed to make your skin feel baby soft. Get creative with these body-buttery bath treats by adding dried flowers. Substitute an infused oil from Chapter 7 for the sweet almond oil to add extra scent and therapeutic value. Make these Bath Melts extra cute by using a decorative mold in the shape of hearts or flowers. A flexible plastic or silicone mold is preferable for this recipe. Package them in decorative glass jars and tie with ribbons for a sweet, homemade gift.

YIELDS: *About 8 (1-ounce) bath melts* *The number of Bath Melts you make depends on what type of mold you use.*

½ cup cocoa butter

¼ cup shea butter

¼ cup sweet almond oil

4 vitamin E capsules

Essential oil blend (see Appendix A)

Dried lavender buds, optional

Dried rose petals, optional

What you will need: double boiler, measuring cups, rubber spatula, ice cube tray, small silicone molds (or loaf pan lined with wax paper) 10–16-ounce glass jar with lid to fit the shape of your melts

① **To Make:** Start the double boiler on medium heat. Once it reaches a boil, reduce heat to simmer. Place the cocoa butter and shea butter in the top of the double boiler and cover. Simmer until melted, stirring occasionally. To preserve the beneficial botanicals, do not overheat. Remove from heat, take the top pan off the double boiler, wipe the water off, and let cool 5–10 minutes. Add the sweet almond oil. Pierce the vitamin E capsules and squeeze the liquid out into the melted oil, discarding the gel caps. Add the essential oils and stir well, scraping any of the hardened cooled mixture off the sides and back into the melted oils. If the mixture hardens too much before you can pour it, gently melt it again in the double boiler. If adding decorative flowers, put a few petals in the bottom of the molds. This will be the top of the melt and the petals will look pretty through the solid butter. Pour the melted butter into your molds, cover with plastic wrap, and let stand undisturbed for 4 hours or overnight. Expedite the solidification process by placing the molds in the refrigerator. The surface will become uneven if they're bumped or moved as they cool, so keep it to a minimum and move them directly after pouring.

2   **To Store:** Carefully remove the Bath Melts from your molds. If they stick, carefully warm the bottom of the mold in hot water. Dry it off before removing because you don't want water on these yet. If you used the loaf pan, remove by pulling up the wax paper. Remove the wax paper, placing the brick of butter on a cutting board. Warm a large knife under hot water and wipe it dry. Cut into 1" cubes. Store the Bath Melts in a sealed container labeled with contents and expiration date of 1–1½ years.

3   **To Use:** Simply drop one Bath Melt into a hot bath for a luxurious moisturizing treat.

SKIN CARE SECRETS

Bathing in hot water causes your body to sweat out toxins, which means that you need to take extra special care to not become dehydrated. Drink lots of fresh water or one of the spa waters found in Chapter 8 to aid the elimination of toxins. Keep in mind that sodas, juices, or even herbal teas are not proper substitutes for good clean water. Your cells need fresh water to keep clean! The more water you drink, the better all of your bodily systems will function, including your skin.

Moisturizing BATH SALTS

It is important to use solar-dried sea salts for your recipes rather than table salt. Naturally dried salts retain the rich vitamins, minerals, trace elements, and amino acids of the sea. Sea salts have a very high concentration of calcium, magnesium, potassium, sodium, and bromide, minerals essential for healthy-looking skin. These minerals are essential for healthy skin and naturally alleviate redness, irritation, and swelling, especially in blemished skin. Soaking in mineral-rich sea salts extracts toxins from your body and relaxes your muscles. So enjoy a long moisturizing soak in these replenishing bath salts!

YIELDS: *1 pint*

1¾ cups solar-dried sea salt

¼ cup sweet almond oil

Essential oil blend (see Appendix A)

What you will need: mixing bowl, spoon, pint jar with lid

1 **To Make:** Place the salt in the bowl. Stir in the sweet almond oil in intervals. Add a little, stir, add a little more, stir, until all of the oil is mixed into the salt. Do the same with the essential oils. Add a little, stir, add a little more, stir, until all of the essential oils are mixed into the salt.

2 **To Store:** Store in a sealed jar labeled with contents and expiration date of 6 months.

3 **To Use:** Draw a bath. When the tub is full, add the bath salts to the water and swish around. Get in the tub and soak for at least 20 minutes, or longer to enjoy maximum therapeutic benefits of the active botanical ingredients. When you are finished soaking, rinse off in the shower to remove the sweat and toxins you released as you bathed. After a bath is also the perfect time to use a body scrub (see Chapter 4), as your skin is softened and easily exfoliated. Follow with moisturizer if desired.

Bath FIZZIES

Bath Fizzies are a fun and effervescent bath treat. Have fun customizing these skin-softening fizzy bath treats by adding dried flowers or substituting extra-virgin coconut oil for the cocoa butter. Make them extra cute by using decorative molds in the shape of hearts or flowers. This recipe will work with metal, plastic, or silicone molds. Package them in decorative glass jars and tie with ribbons for an extra-special homemade gift.

YIELDS: *20 ounces*

The number of Bath Fizzies you make depends on what type of mold you use.

¼ cup cocoa butter

1 cup baking soda

½ cup citric acid

¼ cup cornstarch

½ cup fine-grained sea salt

2 x essential oil blend (see Appendix A)

Dried rose petals, optional

Dried lavender buds, optional

Witch hazel

What you will need: double boiler, rubber gloves, face mask, measuring cups, mixing bowl, sifter or sieve, wooden spoon, spray bottle, small silicone molds or ice cube tray

1 **To Make:** Start the double boiler on medium heat. Once it reaches a boil, reduce heat to simmer. Place the cocoa butter in the top of the double boiler and cover. Simmer until melted, stirring occasionally. To preserve the beneficial botanicals, do not overheat. Remove from heat, take the top pan off the double boiler, and wipe the water off of the bottom. Put on the protective rubber gloves and face mask. Carefully place the baking soda, citric acid, cornstarch, and salt into the sifter. Sift the dry ingredients into the mixing bowl. Carefully stir the powders a little. Add the melted cocoa butter a little at a time, stirring in between. Next, add the essential oils a little at a time, stirring in between. For this recipe, you will need to double the essential oil blend recipes in Appendix A. Break up any clumps with the back of the spoon. If adding decorative flowers, prepare the molds ahead of time by putting a few petals in the bottom of the molds. This will be the top of the fizzie and the petals will make a pretty decoration.

(continued on the following pages)

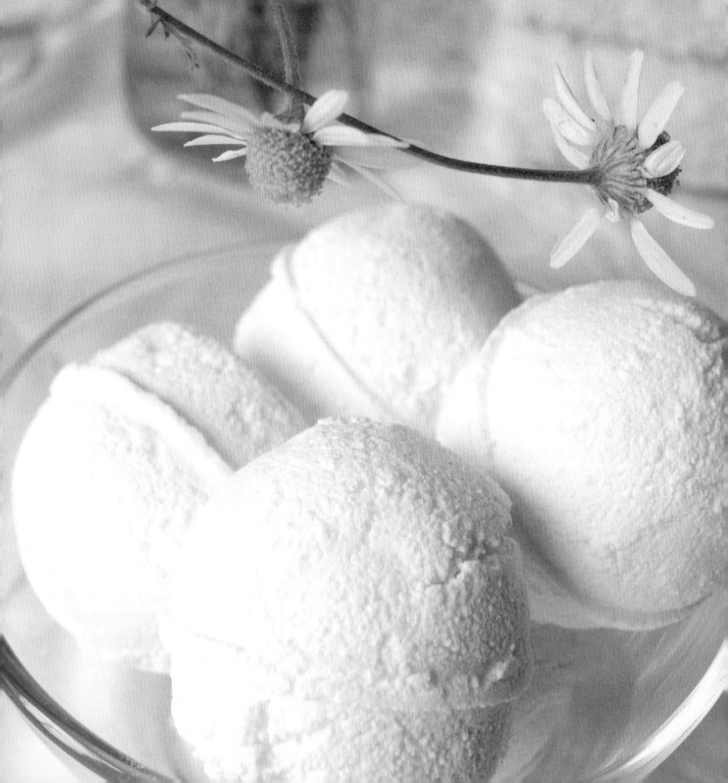

2 Put the witch hazel into the spray bottle. I prefer to mix this stage with my hands (in gloves) like you would a pie crust, but you can also use a wooden spoon. Spray a little at a time—5–6 spritzes—into the fizzie mixture and mix well in between. Repeat this process until the mixture has become moist enough to hold a shape when pressed together, but not wet enough to start fizzing. You want to be careful not to get the mixture too wet, as this activates the fizz. If you hear it start to fizz, stop spraying and mix together. Press tightly into the molds and set out to dry. Let stand for 4 hours or overnight, until completely dry and hardened.

3 **To Store:** Carefully remove the Bath Fizzies from your molds. Store the Bath Fizzies in a sealed container labeled with contents and expiration date of 1–1½ years.

4 **To Use:** Simply drop 1–2 Bath Fizzies into a hot bath for a fun, effervescent, moisturizing treat.

SKIN CARE SECRETS

Using essential oils in the bath is a wonderfully healing aromatherapy experience where gorgeous scent combines with therapeutic effects. As soon as you add the products to the bathwater, the essential oils begin evaporating into the air. To get the most benefit from the essential oils, add your goodies to the tub right before you get in and the healing botanicals will be in full strength to work their magic.

Angel Soak
FOR COLD AND FLU

This all-natural, therapeutic bath soak helps to relieve symptoms such as congestion, body aches, chills, sore throat, headaches, tension, stiffness, and many other signs of common colds and flus. The spices and the heat of the bath will make you sweat, in a good way! The sweating draws out toxins, pollutants, and impurities from your body. The detoxification process will continue after the bath, so be sure to drink lots of healthy fluids and pure clean water. This bath will also help relieve dry, itchy skin. This batch is large enough so you can have it on hand for the cold and flu season!

YIELDS: *1 quart*

4 cups Epsom salts

⅓ cup ground ginger

1½ teaspoons ground cloves

1½ teaspoons ground cinnamon

⅓ cup sweet almond oil

18 drops eucalyptus essential oil

14 drops peppermint essential oil

What you will need: measuring cups and spoons, mixing bowl, wooden spoon, 2 pint jars or 1 quart jar with lid

❶ To Make: Place the Epsom salts, ginger, cloves, and cinnamon in the mixing bowl and stir together with the spoon. Thoroughly disperse the ground spices throughout the salt. Add the sweet almond oil a little at a time, stirring in between. Next, add the essential oils a little at a time, stirring in between. Break up any oily clumps with the back of the spoon, stirring until a uniform blend has been achieved.

❷ To Store: Put the mixture into your jars, label with an expiration date of 1 year, and cap tightly.

❸ To Use: Fill your tub with comfortably hot water or warm-to-lukewarm water, if you have a fever. Add ½ cup of Angel Soak for Cold and Flu to your bath. Soak for at least 20 minutes, or longer. When you are finished soaking, rinse off in the shower to remove the sweat and toxins you released as you bathed. Wrap yourself in a nice warm robe or blanket so that you can continue to sweat it out. Drink a big glass of water and/or a cup of tea and put on some warm socks. Relax, knowing you are on the road to recovery.

SKIN CARE SECRETS

As with all body care products, avoid getting the Angel Soak in your eyes. If this occurs, rinse thoroughly with water. When feeling under the weather, drink warm herbal tea with ginger and lemon to further open nasal passages, and get plenty of rest. This bath should not take the place of qualified medical diagnosis or treatment, nor is it meant to cure any disease or medical condition.

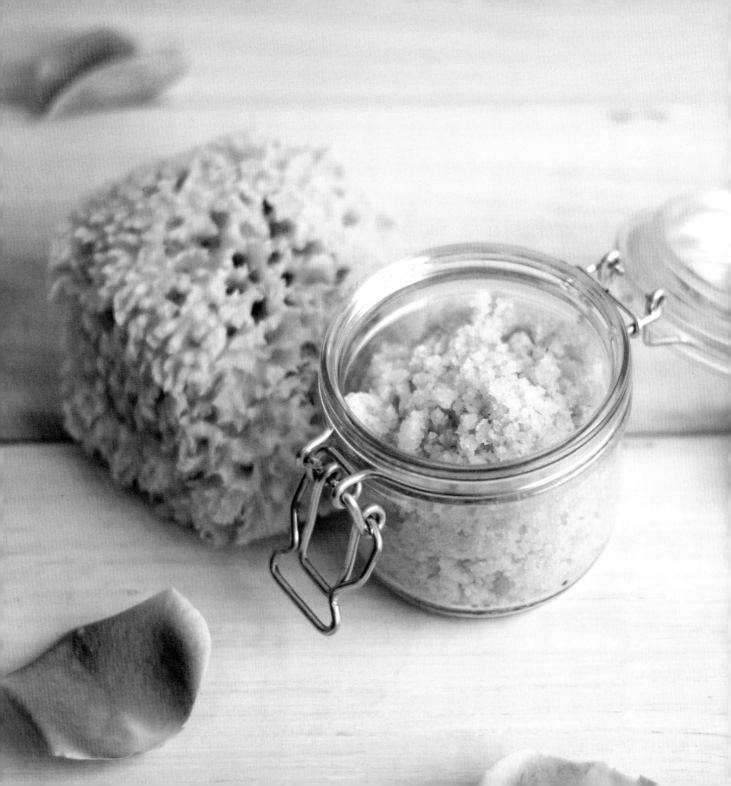

Ideal Luxury BATH

Covet your bath time as an opportunity to celebrate yourself as a fanciful creature of mood, whim, and decadence! This luxurious bath salt blend is rich in sea minerals, Epsom salts, skin-softening sweet almond oil, and skin-conditioning oats. Find your favorite bath combinations by using an infused oil (see Chapter 7) to add scent and therapeutic properties, selecting your favorite essential oil blend (see Appendix A), and using the list of optional additions to make each bath time special and unique according to your ever-changing moods.

YIELDS: *1 quart*

2 cups solar-dried sea salt

¼ cup sweet almond oil or infused oil of choice (see Chapter 7)

½ cup baking soda

¼ cup oat flour

1 cup Epsom salts

2 x essential oil blend (see Appendix A)

What you will need: mixing bowl, spoon, quart jar with lid

❶ To Make: Place the sea salt in the bowl and stir in the sweet almond oil. Next, blend in the baking soda, oat flour, and Epsom salts. Add the essential oils in intervals, stirring in between, until all of the essential oils are mixed into the salts.

❷ To Store: Store in a sealed jar labeled with contents and expiration date of 6 months.

❸ To Use: Draw a bath. When the tub is full, add ¼ cup or the desired amount of bath salts to the water and swish around. Add any optional embellishments from the sidebar on the following page. Get in the tub and soak for at least 20 minutes, or longer to enjoy maximum therapeutic benefits of the active botanical ingredients. When you are finished soaking, rinse off in the shower to remove the sweat and toxins you released as you bathed. After a bath is also the perfect time to use a body scrub (see Chapter 4), as your skin is softened and easily exfoliated. Follow with moisturizer if desired.

(continued on the following page)

SKIN CARE SECRETS

To make your bath extra special, add a scoop of Ideal Luxury Bath blend to the water and supplement one or more ingredients from the list below. Note: The following additions are meant as a per-bath addition and should not be incorporated into the recipe on page 123.

- 1 cup full-fat milk (soy, coconut, or dairy)
- 1 cup yogurt
- Petals from a blooming rose or other edible flowers
- ¼ cup honey
- Fresh citrus slices
- ¼ cup cocoa powder
- Sachet of fresh or dried herbs or flowers: lavender, chamomile, comfrey, red clover, calendula, witch hazel, lemongrass, hibiscus, echinacea, mint, or rose petals

Chamomile and Oat
SUPER SOOTHE-ME BATH

Oatmeal baths are relaxing and soothing, especially for skin that's dry, itchy, or inflamed. This bath helps alleviate the symptoms of skin conditions such as eczema, psoriasis, rashes, allergies, insect bites, chicken pox, sunburn, and more. Chamomile will accentuate the calming effect, leaving you comforted and relaxed in mind, body, and spirit.

YIELDS: *1 quart*

½ cup sweet almond oil

1 cup baking soda

2 cups whole oats

¾ cup dried chamomile flowers

¼ cup dried lavender buds

What you will need: measuring cups, large mixing bowl, spoon, quart jar with lid, small muslin drawstring bag

❶ To Make: Mix the sweet almond oil and baking soda together in a large bowl. It will be a dry mixture. Add the oats and stir. Add the chamomile and lavender and blend to a uniform consistency.

❷ To Store: Label and store in a tight-sealing jar for up to 6 months.

❸ To Use: Loosely fill the cloth bag with the Chamomile and Oat Super Soothe-Me Bath, making a sachet. Tie a bow tight enough that it won't come apart in use. Remember, you will need to untie it later to clean it out and use it again. Fill the tub with warm water and drop in the sachet. Do not use the sachet to rub irritated skin, but gently squeeze the liquid from the sachet over your body and relax. Dry off with care, using gentle blotting actions with a soft towel over the itchy or sore parts of your skin. Repeat as needed. Oatmeal baths are gentle and can be enjoyed every day.

(continued on the following page)

SKIN CARE SECRETS

You can also use this Chamomile and Oat Super Soothe-Me Bath to make bath sachets for party favors or gifts. Put about ½ cup of the mixture in the center of a piece of cloth and close tightly with a rubber band or piece of string. Tie a ribbon around it to make it pretty. You can use small cloth bags for the sachets. Package into individual cello bags, and tie closed to retain freshness. Add a label that says "Soothing Bath Sachet" with instructions for use and a "use by" date.

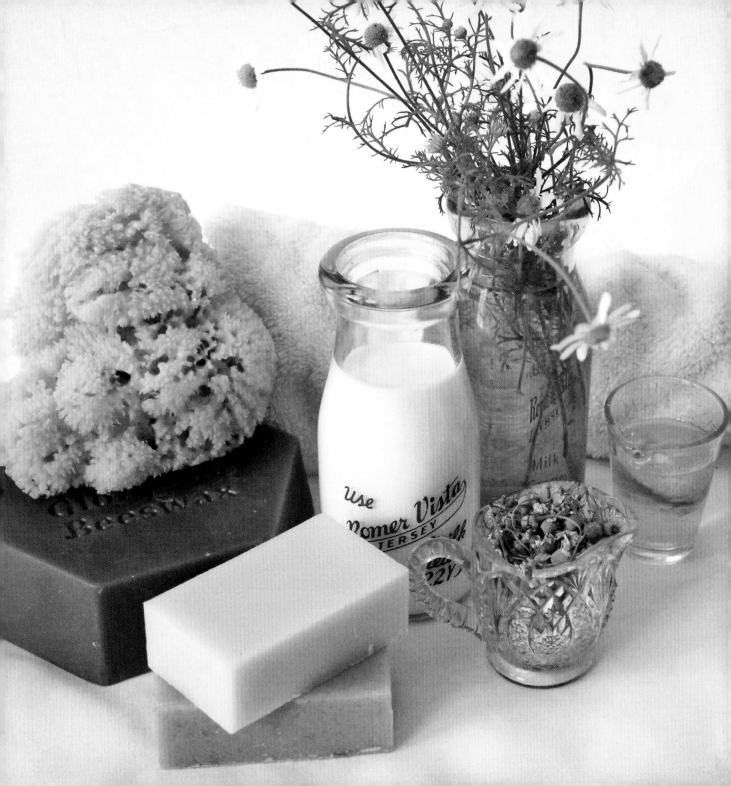

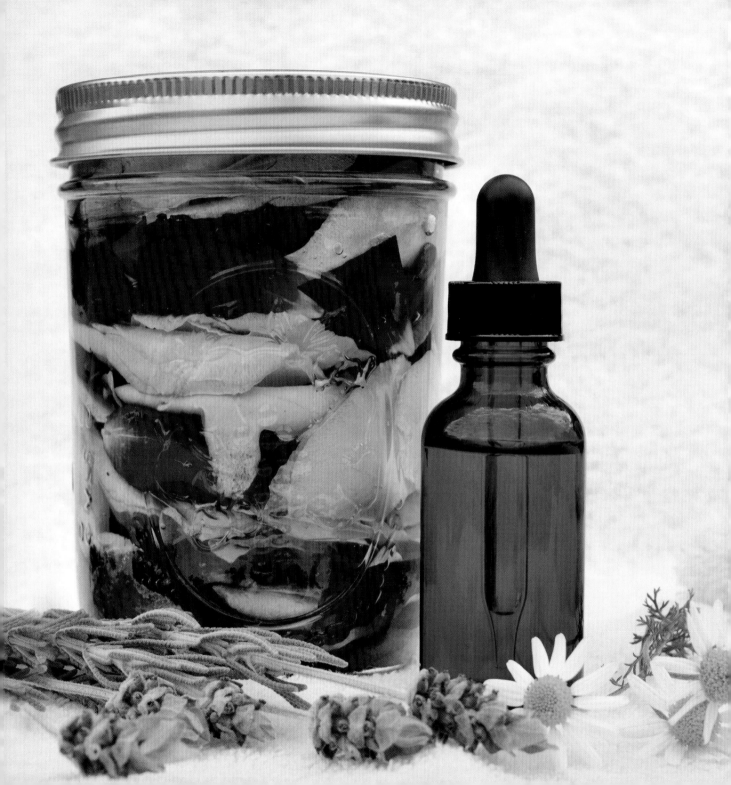

CHAPTER 7

INFUSIONS

Herbal infusions have been used for centuries in natural healing. Soaking seeds, flowers, leaves, roots, or bark in liquid is a time-honored and very easy method of transferring the beneficial properties and gorgeous scent (or flavor) of the plant material into a usable medium. You can infuse plant material into alcohol, water, or oil, depending on the type of plant you wish to infuse and the desired application of the finished product. While some infusions in this chapter—like the Old-Fashioned Rosewater and the Layered Lavender Flower Water—will be made with water, the majority will be made with oil. We recommend using jojoba oil for the oil infusions, as it works well in all skin care recipes, can withstand sustained heat if required, and has a comparatively long shelf life of two years or more. If you'd like, you can substitute another carrier oil (base oil) for the jojoba, but this will lessen the infusion's shelf life to that of the carrier oil you choose.

All of the infusions in this chapter can be safely used on the skin in a variety of preparations without being diluted like essential oils, and they are incorporated as ingredients into various recipes throughout the book. The infused oil will have both the properties of its carrier oil and the properties of the plants that were used in the infusion. Use these gorgeous infusions daily in your skin care regimen for face and body and have fun creatively incorporating them into the fabulous spa products you make from this book. Your artisan infusions will also make beautiful handmade gifts for family and friends.

Green Tea-Infused OIL

Green tea has tremendous benefits as a skin care ingredient. It has been shown to reactivate dying skin cells, thereby improving the condition of the skin. This nourishing antioxidant-rich all-purpose oil is used as a base ingredient in several recipes throughout the book, but you can also use it on its own as an anti-aging oil for your face and body.

YIELDS: *8 ounces*

½ cup loose-leaf green tea

1 cup jojoba oil or coconut oil (coconut oil is solid at 76°F (24.4°C); use coconut oil for this infusion as a stand-alone body butter in cooler climates)

What you will need: double boiler, measuring cups, rubber spatula, strainer (cheesecloth or tea strainer), 8-ounce bottle or jar, funnel

1 **To Make:** Start a double boiler on medium heat. Once boiling, reduce heat to a simmer. Place the green tea into the top of the double boiler. If using jojoba oil, pour it over the tea leaves, saturating them. If using coconut oil, melt it first in the double boiler and then add the green tea, stirring to saturate the leaves. Cover and simmer on low heat for 1 hour. Check back every 20 minutes or so to make sure there is enough water in the double boiler. Remove from heat, take the top pot off the double boiler, and let cool.

2 **To Store:** Strain tea from oil into a storage jar. The jojoba will remain liquid. Place the coconut oil in the refrigerator to cool and solidify back to a solid butter form. Will keep 2 years or longer if stored in a cool dark place.

3 **To Use:** For use as a facial moisturizing oil: Mist your face with Old-Fashioned Rosewater (see page 145) or your favorite toner. Place a few drops of Green Tea-Infused Oil onto the tips of your fingers and gently massage the oil into your facial skin.

HELPFUL HINTS

Jojoba oil and coconut oil are specified for this recipe because both of these oils have a relatively long shelf life and are particularly beneficial for facial care use. However, they are not interchangeable when specified in the recipes throughout this book due to the drastic difference in consistency. Jojoba oil is liquid and coconut oil is solid at 76°F (24.4°C). For example, the green tea-infused jojoba is used in the Vital Facial Moisturizer and coconut oil is called for in the Green Tea Eye Cream (see Chapter 2). Keeping this in mind, you can also substitute your favorite carrier oil to suit your needs.

Chai Spice-Infused OIL

This exotic scented oil makes a fantastic bath, body, or massage oil and is used as a base ingredient for the Sugar Chai Honey Scrub (Chapter 4). The warming, antioxidant-rich chai spices include cinnamon, cardamom, nutmeg, star anise, ginger, fennel, and black pepper, along with black tea. In Ayurvedic traditions, chai spices are known to be calming, vitalizing, and mentally clarifying. Get ready for your house to smell really, really good.

YIELDS: *8 ounces*

8 ounces jojoba oil

½ cup loose chai tea

4 vitamin E capsules

What you will need: double boiler, measuring cups, rubber spatula, strainer (cheesecloth or tea strainer), dark-colored 8-ounce bottle, funnel.

❶ **To Make:** Start a double boiler on medium heat. Once boiling, reduce heat to a simmer. Place the chai spices into the pan. Pour the jojoba oil over the spices, saturating them. Cover and simmer on low heat for 1 hour. Check back every 20 minutes or so to make sure there is enough water in the double boiler. Remove from heat, take the top pot off the double boiler, and let cool. Strain the tea from the oil into a bottle. Pierce the vitamin E capsules and squeeze the liquid out into the bottle, discarding the gel caps. Place cap on tightly and shake well to blend.

❷ **To Store:** Will keep up to 2 years if stored out of direct sunlight.

❸ **To Use:** Use as an exotic bath, body, or massage oil.

Rosemary-Infused OIL

"There's rosemary, that's for remembrance; pray, love, remember . . ." says Ophelia in Shakespeare's *Hamlet*. And it's true! Ancient Greek students wore a wreath of rosemary around their heads while studying. Rosemary has long been known to stimulate the conscious mind, keeping one alert and calm. Herbal healers have also used rosemary since ancient times to help relieve a plethora of ailments, including arthritis, headaches, muscle spasms, and cold and flu symptoms. It also soothes itchy skin, conditions the hair and scalp, and is beneficial in the treatment of cellulite.

YIELDS: *8 ounces*

½ cup rosemary (fresh or dried)

8 ounces jojoba oil

4 vitamin E capsules

What you will need: double boiler, measuring cups, rubber spatula, strainer (cheesecloth or tea strainer), 8-ounce bottle or jar (preferably dark colored), funnel

❶ **To Make:** Start a double boiler on medium heat. Once boiling, reduce heat to a simmer. Place the rosemary into the pan. Pour in the jojoba oil, saturating the rosemary. Cover and simmer on low heat for 1 hour. Check back every 20 minutes or so to make sure there is enough water in the double boiler. Remove from heat, take the top pot off the double boiler, wipe dry with a towel, and let cool. Strain the herb from the oil into an 8-ounce Mason jar or bottle. Pierce the vitamin E capsules and squeeze the liquid out into the bottle, discarding the gel caps. Place cap on tightly and shake well to blend.

❷ **To Store:** Store in a cool dry place out of direct sunlight. Will keep up to 2 years, or longer if kept in the fridge.

❸ **To Use:** This infusion can be used as is for massage or bathing, or as a body oil to relieve any of the symptoms listed above, and is an active ingredient in recipes throughout this book.

(continued on the following page)

HELPFUL HINTS

Throughout this chapter, you'll find recipes that call for fresh herbs, dried herbs, or either of the two. For all of these recipes, if you plan to use fresh, buy or pick them a day or two ahead of time and set them out to wilt overnight to reduce some of the water content. Pick from the garden after the morning dew has dried, or buy organic nonsprayed herbs from the farmers' market. It's best not to wash the leaves to help prevent mildew. If you need to wash them, make sure they dry thoroughly before preparing the recipes. To dry, lay them out on dish towels or string a line in your pantry and hang them with clothespins overnight. Do not leave them in the sun. Additionally, if you remove the leaves from the stems when they are freshly picked, the herb will retain more of the vital nutrients, increasing the beneficial properties of the infusion.

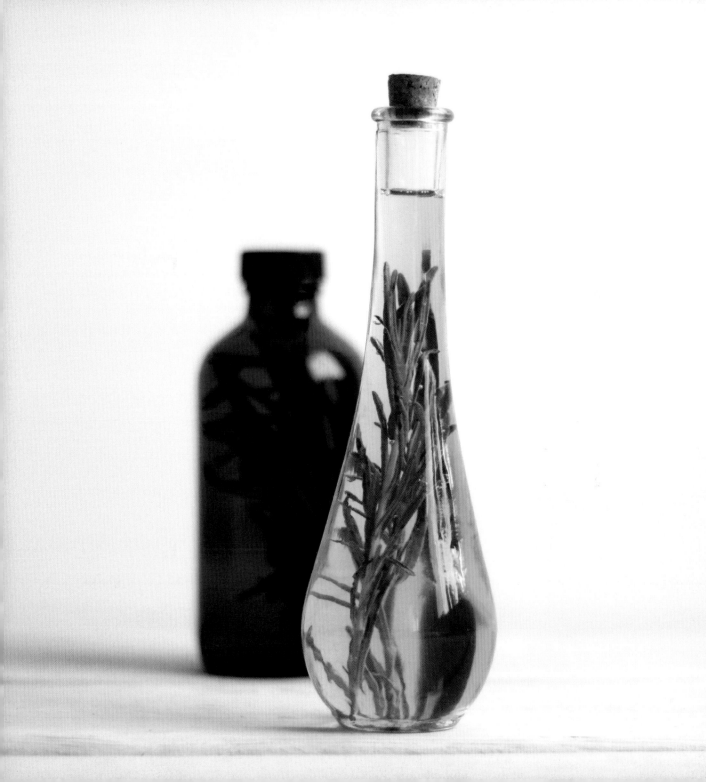

Vanilla-Infused OIL

Is there any scent more universally loved than vanilla? Vanilla-Infused Oil can be used as the base oil for several recipes throughout the book——including the Vanilla, Bourbon, and Honey Scrub (Chapter 4)——and you can also use this infusion as is for a lovely bath, body, or massage oil.

YIELDS: *8 ounces*

8 ounces jojoba oil or carrier oil of choice

2–3 vanilla beans

4 vitamin E capsules

What you will need: double boiler, measuring cups, paring knife, rubber spatula, strainer (cheesecloth or tea strainer), 8-ounce bottle, funnel

❶ **To Make:** Start a double boiler on medium heat. Once boiling, reduce heat to a low simmer. Put the jojoba oil in the top of the double boiler. With a sharp knife, slice the vanilla beans lengthwise and scrape out the seeds with the edge of the knife. Put the seeds into the pan of oil. Chop the vanilla pods into small pieces and put into the oil. Cover and let simmer for at least an hour. You can simmer this concoction for as long as you like. The longer, the better, actually, but remember to check back every 20 minutes or so to make sure there is enough water in the double boiler. Remove from heat, take the top pot off the double boiler, and let cool. Pour oil, without straining, into an 8-ounce bottle. Pierce the vitamin E capsules and squeeze the liquid out into the bottle, discarding the gel caps. Place cap on tightly and shake well to blend.

❷ **To Store:** Will keep 2 years or longer if stored in the bottle in a cool dark place out of direct sunlight.

❸ **To Use:** Use as a moisturizer, massage oil, or add a couple of teaspoons to your bathwater for a vanilla-infused moisture bath.

HELPFUL HINTS

I leave the vanilla bits in the bottle so they can continue to impart their magic to the oil. If you prefer, strain the mixture before pouring into your container. The small vanilla seeds will remain in the oil, but they're beneficial in the body scrub recipes.

Fresh Comfrey OIL

Comfrey is widely known as one of nature's greatest medicinal herbs, so this infusion will make an excellent addition to your healing toolbox. Comfrey is an excellent herb to add to boost the therapeutic anti-inflammatory and overall healing properties of natural skin care products. Use it to heal bruises, burns, rashes, and more. This recipe is especially beneficial for all manner of skin conditions, including eczema and psoriasis.

YIELDS: *9 ounces*

1 cup fresh comfrey leaves

1 cup jojoba oil

4 vitamin E capsules

What you will need: quart jar, dark-colored 8-ounce bottle, strainer (cheesecloth or tea strainer), chopstick

❶ **To Make:** Finely chop the comfrey leaves and place in the quart jar. Cover the plant matter completely with jojoba oil. Stir well with the chopstick to remove any air bubbles and completely saturate the plant material. To avoid oxidation and spoilage of the fresh herb, leave as little air space as possible in the jar. Top off with more oil if necessary and tightly close the lid. Label the jar with the date and contents and place in a warm dark place to infuse for 2–4 weeks. Shake well each day. After 2–4 weeks, strain the herb from the oil into a sterilized 8-ounce bottle. Do not squeeze out the herb to avoid getting juice from the comfrey into the oil. Pierce the vitamin E capsules and squeeze the liquid out into the bottle, discarding the gel caps. Place cap on tightly and shake well to blend. Check back on this infusion after a week to see if any juice has settled in the oil. If so, decant it out and place the oil into a clean dry jar.

❷ **To Store:** Label the bottle with contents and expiration date of 1 year. Store in a cool dry place out of direct sunlight.

❸ **To Use:** Use as a bath, body, or massage oil.

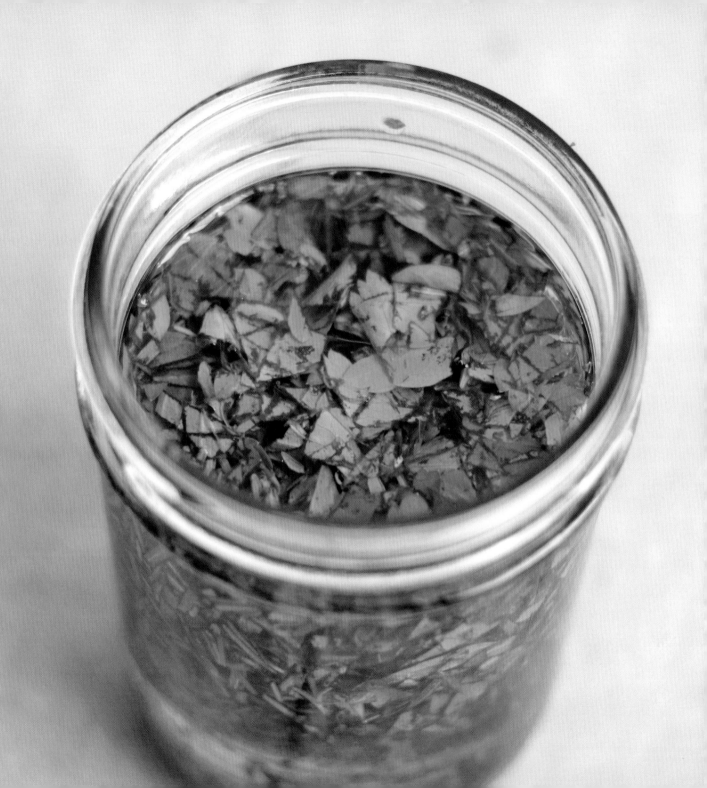

Fresh HERBAL OIL

This refreshing garden herb-scented blend is beneficial for sore muscles, respiratory health, and antibacterial skin care needs. The antibacterial herbs thyme, rosemary, oregano, and parsley also boost circulation, and the marjoram used here is warming and comforting.

YIELDS: *about 8 ounces*

⅛ cup fresh thyme leaves

¼ cup fresh rosemary leaves

¼ cup fresh oregano leaves

¼ cup fresh parsley leaves

⅛ cup fresh marjoram leaves

9 ounces jojoba oil

4 vitamin E capsules

What you will need: measuring cups, mixing bowl, strainer (cheesecloth or tea strainer), 16-ounce (pint-size) canning jar, funnel, dark-colored 8-ounce bottle

1 **To Make:** Crush all of the herbs slightly and place them into the 16-ounce jar. Pour the jojoba oil over the herbs, saturating them. Close the lid tightly and shake, thoroughly saturating the herbs in the oil. Top off with more oil if necessary, replacing the lid tightly. Store in a warm dark place for at least 30 days and up to 60 days. Shake the jar daily to keep the infusion active, but keep it closed. Strain the plant material from the oil into an 8-ounce bottle. Pierce the vitamin E capsules and squeeze the liquid out into the bottle, discarding the gel caps. Place cap on tightly and shake well to blend.

2 **To Store:** Will remain potent for up to 2 years if stored in a cool dark place. Lengthen the shelf life by storing in the refrigerator. The oil will become thick and cloudy when cold, but will warm back up to liquid when left at room temperature for 30 minutes or so.

3 **To Use:** Can be used as an herbal scented bath, body, or massage oil.

Lavender-Infused OIL

Lavender's aroma is simultaneously stimulating and relaxing. It has been known to help a headache and ease muscular pain and respiratory ailments. Lavender soothes and calms the skin, balances oil production, speeds healing of scars and blemishes, and stimulates circulation for improved skin tone. Lavender is associated with the third-eye chakra, whose attributes include intuition, imagination, visualization, and concentration. Lavender-Infused Oil is a gorgeous multipurpose universal healing elixir for mind, body, and spirit.

YIELDS: *8 ounces*

1 cup fresh or dried lavender flowers
8 ounces jojoba oil or carrier oil of choice
4 vitamin E capsules

What you will need: quart jar, measuring cups, chopstick, strainer (cheesecloth or tea strainer), 8-ounce bottle, funnel

❶ To Make: If using fresh lavender, coarsely chop the buds and place in the quart jar. If using dried lavender, crush slightly with your hand as you put the buds into the jar. Cover the plant matter completely with jojoba oil. Stir well with the chopstick to remove any air bubbles and completely saturate the plant material. To avoid oxidation and spoilage of the fresh herb, leave as little air space as possible in the jar. Top off with more oil if necessary and tightly close the lid. Label the jar with the date and contents and place in a warm dark place to infuse for 2–4 weeks. Shake the jar daily. After 2–4 weeks, strain the herb from the oil into a sterilized 8-ounce bottle. Pierce the vitamin E capsules and squeeze the liquid out into the bottle, discarding the gel caps. Place cap on tightly and shake well to blend. If you used fresh lavender flowers, check back on this infusion after a week to see if any plant juice has settled in the oil. If so, decant it out and place the oil into a clean dry bottle.

❷ To Store: Label the bottle with contents and expiration date of 2 years. If you substituted another oil for the jojoba oil, adjust the expiration date to the shelf life of the oil used. Store in a cool dry place out of direct sunlight.

❸ To Use: Makes a fantastic bath, body, or massage oil; see above for indications.

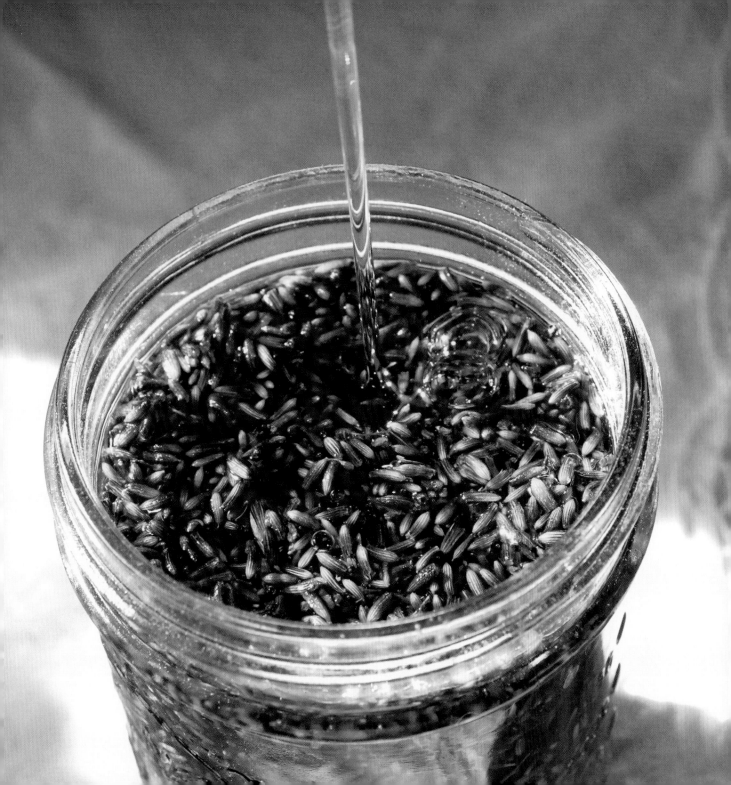

Sweet Dreamtime–Infused OIL

This sweet, dreamily scented oil is a calming, relaxing blend of botanicals to promote peaceful and restful sleep. Sweet Dreamtime–Infused Oil makes the perfect spa product for helping you relax before bed, soothing your senses with a botanical lullaby. Use fresh or dried herbs depending on availability.

YIELDS: *8 ounces*

¼ cup marjoram

¼ cup lavender buds

½ cup chamomile flowers

8 ounces jojoba oil

4 vitamin E capsules

What you will need: quart-size jar, measuring cups, chopstick, strainer (cheesecloth or tea strainer), dark-colored 8-ounce bottle, funnel

1 **To Make:** If using fresh herbs, coarsely chop them and place in the quart-size jar. If using dried herbs, crush slightly with your hand as you put the plant material into the jar. Cover the plant matter completely with jojoba oil. Stir well with the chopstick to remove any air bubbles and completely saturate the plant material. To avoid oxidation and spoilage of fresh herbs and to maximize your infusion, leave as little air space as possible in the jar. Top off with more oil if necessary and tightly close the lid. Label the jar with the date and contents and place in a warm dark place to infuse for 2–4 weeks. Shake the jar daily. After 2–4 weeks, strain the herb from the oil into a sterilized 8-ounce bottle. Pierce the vitamin E capsules and squeeze the liquid out into the bottle, discarding the gel caps. Place cap on tightly and shake well to blend. If you used fresh herbs, check back on this infusion after a week to see if any plant juice has settled in the oil. If so, decant it out and place the oil into a clean dry jar.

2 **To Store:** Label the bottle with contents and expiration date of 2 years. If you substituted another oil for the jojoba oil, adjust the expiration date to the shelf life of the oil used. Store in a cool dry place out of direct sunlight.

3 **To Use:** Use as bath, body, or massage oil, specifically before bedtime or when relaxation is desired.

Layered
LAVENDER FLOWER WATER

Lavender is a universal healer for your mind, body, and spirit. This Layered Lavender Flower Water is relaxing and balancing for the skin, and it makes a fantastic toner for all skin types, especially oily and combination skin. You can also add it to your bath water for a tranquil soak or put it in a spray bottle and spritz to cool down on a hot day. A little spritz of lavender water can help ease a hot flash, soothe a sunburn, or calm itchy skin, or you can use it as a linen spray right before climbing into bed for a calming drift off into dreamland.

YIELDS: *16 ounces*

2 cups distilled water

½ cup dried lavender flowers or 1 cup fresh flowers (stems removed)

¼ cup witch hazel

60 drops lavender essential oil

What you will need: glass or enamel pot, strainer (cheesecloth or tea strainer), funnel jar or bottle with sprayer top (optional) to hold 16 ounces

❶ **To Make:** Boil the water and pour over the lavender flowers. Steep for 20–30 minutes. While the lavender is brewing, put the witch hazel into your storage container and add essential oil. When the lavender brew is ready, strain it into the bottle. Place the cap on and shake well to blend the ingredients.

❷ **To Store:** Store bottle in your refrigerator for up to 6 months.

❸ **To Use:** Shake well before each use. Use as a facial toner or as an aromatic body, hair, linen, or room spray.

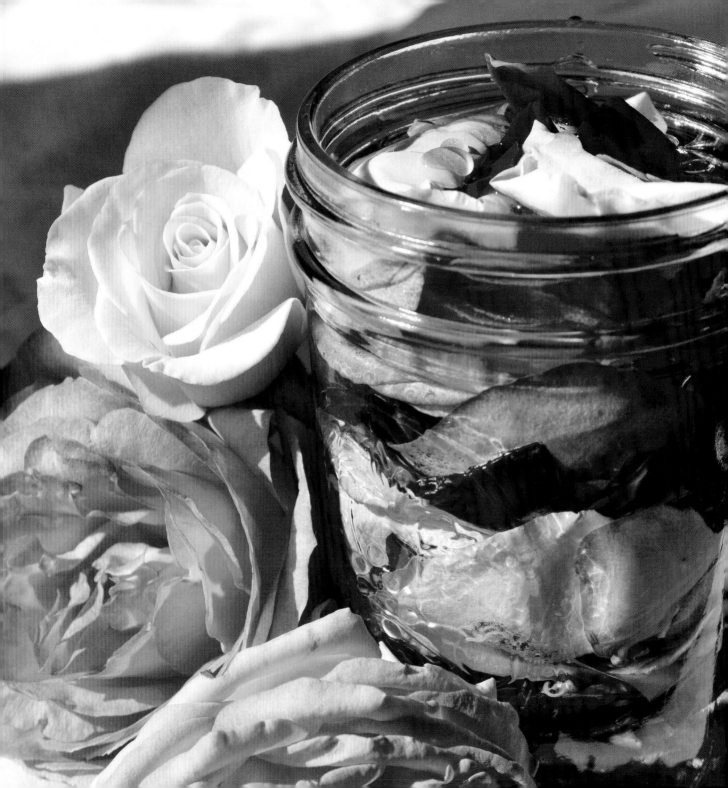

Old-Fashioned ROSEWATER

Rosewater is truly a nectar of the gods. It can be used in many recipes, from foods to beauty aids, or just be splashed on for a fragrant aura as lovely as a rose! Rosewater also makes a wonderful facial toner for all skin types and is used in several recipes throughout this book, including the Rooibos Rose Toner (Chapter 2) and the Green Clay Rose Milk Mask (Chapter 3).

YIELDS: *16 ounces*

2 cups rose petals

2 cups distilled water

Dash of sea salt

What you will need: rubber gloves, glass or enamel pot, strainer (cheesecloth or tea strainer), funnel, jar or bottle with sprayer top (optional) to hold 16 ounces

❶ **To Make:** Place the rose petals in a glass or enamel pot, pour in distilled water to just cover. Avoid using a metal pot, as it will react negatively with the oils. Add a dash of sea salt to help bring the essential oils out of the petals. Heat until water is scalding but not boiling. Turn off the heat, add rose petals, and let soak for at least an hour. Strain the petals from the liquid, and use the funnel to pour into your storage container. Wear rubber gloves to help avoid contamination, and give the petals an extra squeeze to get as much of the botanical goodness out of them as possible.

❷ **To Store:** Store in your refrigerator for up to 4 months.

❸ **To Use:** Use as a facial toner or add a cup to your bathwater along with a few fresh rose petals for a delicate rosy bath. Makes a lovely aromatic mist to refresh your skin and your spirits if kept in a bottle with a sprayer top.

SKIN CARE SECRETS

Traditional hydrosols, a.k.a. flower waters, are the by-product of steam distillation of essential oils. Steam passes through the plant material to extract the essential oils; the hydrosol is the condensed steam. Floral waters are much milder than essential oils and have similar therapeutic effects in skin care and in overall mind, body, and spirit wellness.

Aromatic
VANILLA INFUSION

This divinely scented vanilla mist is a gorgeous way to scent your hair and body.
A little spritz of this comforting aphrodisiac scent instantly
sets the mood to cozy and romantic.

YIELDS: *8 ounces*

3 vanilla beans
8 ounces witch hazel

What you will need: cutting board, knife, 8-ounce bottle with cap, funnel

1 **To Make:** Slice the vanilla beans into thin strips and cut into smaller pieces. Place them into the bottle. Fill it up with witch hazel and shake well. Store it in a cool dark place for at least 2 weeks. Ideally you will remember to shake it up daily, but it's okay if you skip a day or 2. The longer you leave the vanilla beans to soak, the stronger your infusion will be. When you've reached your desired strength, strain out the vanilla and use a funnel to pour the brew back into the bottle.

2 **To Store:** Label with expiration date of 2 years and store in a cool dark place out of direct sunlight.

3 **To Use:** Shake well before each use. Use as a facial toner for normal to oily skin or as an aromatic body, hair, linen, or room spray.

SKIN CARE SECRETS

If you plan to use this Aromatic Vanilla Infusion in facial care, consider mixing 1 part aloe vera juice with 3 parts Aromatic Vanilla Infusion for added benefit. Start with a high quality witch hazel, easily found at a health food store or online, that has a higher percentage of witch hazel extract than alcohol.

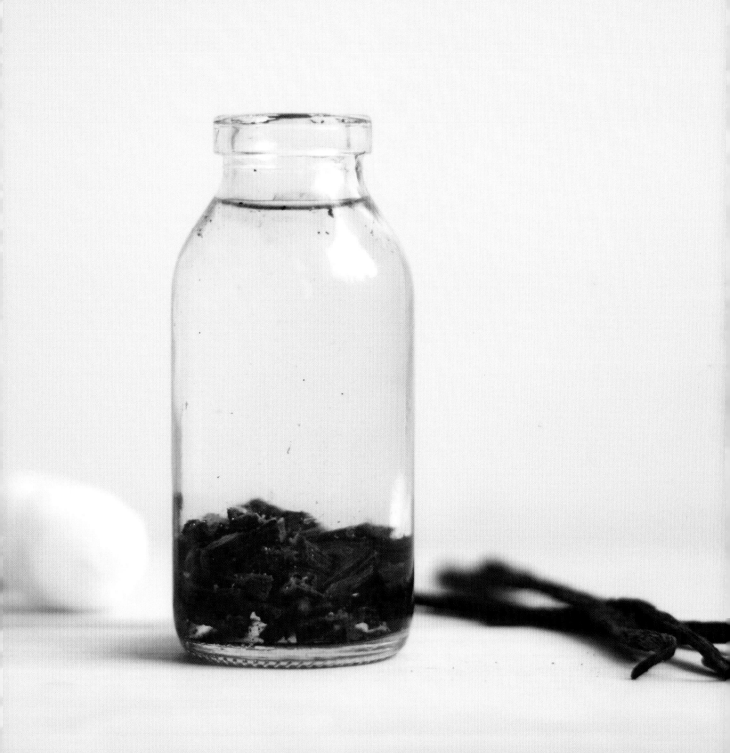

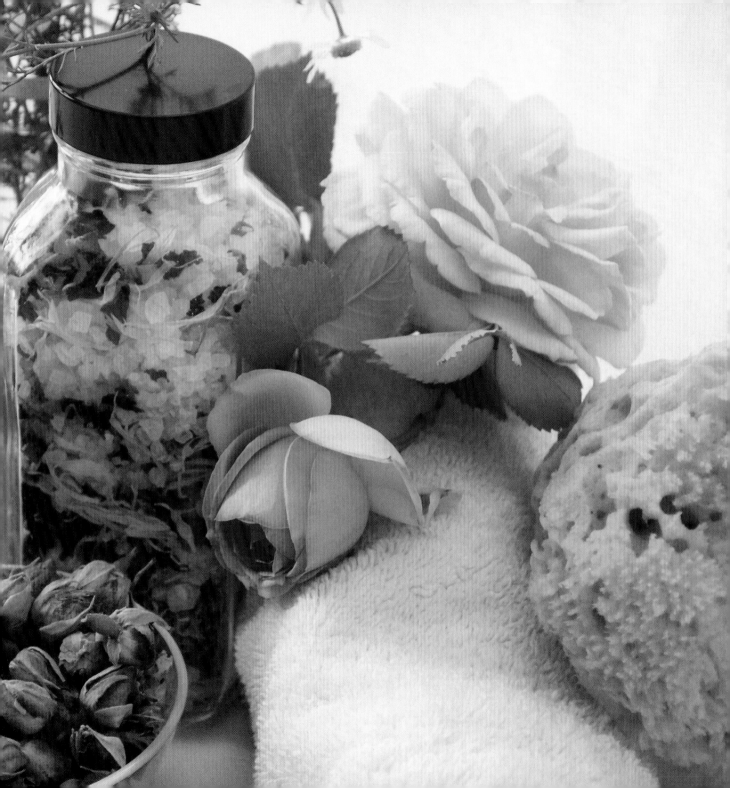

CHAPTER 8

WHOLE-BODY SPA TREATMENTS

Whether you're getting ready for a special event like a wedding or a party or just taking some time to focus on yourself, the recipes in this chapter provide a rich sensory journey to leave you positively glowing from the inside out. Taking the extra time to set the scene for a divine home spa experience brings the pampering to a higher level of replenishment and rejuvenation, nurturing your mind, body, and spirit.

Start by letting fresh air flow through your space to clear out any stagnant energy or stale air. Select some calming, healing music to play. Lay out some clean fluffy towels and a soft robe. In the spirit of whole body replenishment, prepare a healthy spa water like the Strawberry Super C Sipper or Cucumber De-Puffer Spa Water to enjoy while you recline with your feet soaking in a Fizzy Mojito Foot Spa. Light some candles and say a blessing. Something like this works well to set the tone: "I have set this time aside for me. All of my stresses and worries fall away from me now. This is my time to heal and nurture my entire being." Take a few deep breaths to set the relaxation in motion. It is in these sweet moments, while you are in repose slathered in gorgeous, gooey home spa treatments like the Head-to-Toe Pumpkin Mask or the Detoxifying Seaweed Body Wrap, that a deeper overall healing takes place. There is nothing comparable to a spa day like this to bring out your inner goddess!

Head-to-Toe
PUMPKIN MASK

Pumpkin is loaded with more than one-hundred vitamins and nutrients that feed your skin. It's a naturally nourishing, hydrating exfoliant. Paired with the skin-brightening, clarifying orange, soothing oats, and moisturizing olive oil found in this recipe, this mask can be used from head to toe for a gorgeous glow! The active enzymes in the pumpkin may cause a tingling sensation. A slight warming on the skin will be normal due to the fresh ginger and cinnamon.

YIELDS: *1–2 full body masks*

1 cup flesh of 1 small pumpkin, prepared, or
   1 can pumpkin

½ cup cooked oatmeal

¼ teaspoon ground cinnamon

¼ cup extra-virgin olive oil

1 teaspoon fresh grated ginger

½ teaspoon fresh grated orange zest

1 tablespoon fresh-squeezed orange juice

½ cup raw turbinado sugar

① **To Make:** Begin by preparing the fresh pumpkin, or skip this step and use canned. Cut the pumpkin into quarters or medium 3–4-inch chunks, leaving rind on. Place rind-side down (flesh up) in a vegetable steamer. Bring to a boil, reduce heat to simmer, and cover. Steam 10–15 minutes until a fork will easily glide through the chunks, like a cooked potato. Be careful not to overcook, it as it will lose potency. Remove from heat and let cool to the touch. Scoop out the pumpkin flesh with a spoon, discarding the rind. Reserve 1 cup for this recipe and use the remainder for soup, a pie, or custard. Place the prepared pumpkin in the fridge. While the pumpkin is steaming, cook the oatmeal by following the directions on the package. Place the cooked oatmeal in the fridge to ensure it has completely cooled before moving onto the next step. In a medium-size bowl, use a fork to blend together the oatmeal, cinnamon, and olive oil. Let stand for 10–15 minutes and begin preparing the other fresh ingredients. Mash the pumpkin and add to the bowl along with the grated ginger, orange zest, and orange juice and stir to a uniform consistency. Add the sugar and blend well.

② **To Store:** This mask will store in the refrigerator for up to a few days in a clean, airtight container. The pumpkin will oxidize quickly, so it's best to use ultra fresh rather than prepare ahead of your home spa day.

③ **To Use:** For best results, take a quick shower or use after a long soak in the tub to soften your skin and remove surface dirt and toxins. The warmth of the shower will open your pores and the moisture on your skin will provide a conduit for the mask to start working faster and more effectively. Towel dry and apply a generous layer of the mask over your body. You can wrap yourself in a clean sheet or plastic wrap and relax in an empty bath tub, or just sit on your towel. Let the body mask work its magic for 15 minutes, then apply to the face. Leave on the face for 3–7 minutes. Jump in the shower and rinse off. You may want a washcloth to help remove the mask. Use a mild body wash or soap and moisturize with your favorite lotion or body oil.

Glowing Goddess
FACE AND BODY MASK

Cleopatra's favorite beauty treatment was bathing in milk, honey, and roses. This enchanting combination will nourish, moisturize, exfoliate, and invigorate your skin to a gorgeous glow. Use this decadent whole body mask for soft milk-and-honey skin that radiates with a gorgeous goddess glow.

YIELDS: *1–2 full body masks*

Petals of 2 roses
½ cup honey
¾ cup heavy cream (or coconut cream)
1 cup almond meal

What you will need: blender, rubber spatula, mixing bowl, measuring cups, fork

1 **To Make:** Place the rose petals, honey, and cream into the blender and mix on low until you have a uniform blend. Place the creamed roses in the mixing bowl, using the rubber spatula to remove as much as possible from the blender. Add the almond meal and stir with a fork until you have a uniform consistency. Add more cream or almond meal, a little at a time as necessary to achieve a spreadable paste.

2 **To Store:** This is best used fresh. Plan to prepare this recipe just before your spa treatment. Store leftovers in a sealed container in the refrigerator and use up within a day or 2.

3 **To Use:** For best results, take a quick shower or use after a long soak in the tub. The warmth of the shower will open your pores and the moisture on your skin will provide a conduit for the mask to start working faster and more effectively. Towel dry and apply to skin in small, upward motions. Start with your body and finish with your face. Once you are covered from head to toe, massage the scrub in small circular motions, starting with the legs and arms, making your way up to the torso, ending at your heart. Then move to your face, avoiding the eye area. Massage your face with light pressure, using circular motions. Allow to set on your body for up to 30 minutes and up to 15 minutes on your face. To remove, get in the shower and rinse well. For maximum benefit, do not use soap to wash off the residual oils. Towel dry and mist your face with Old-Fashioned Rosewater (see Chapter 7) to close the pores.

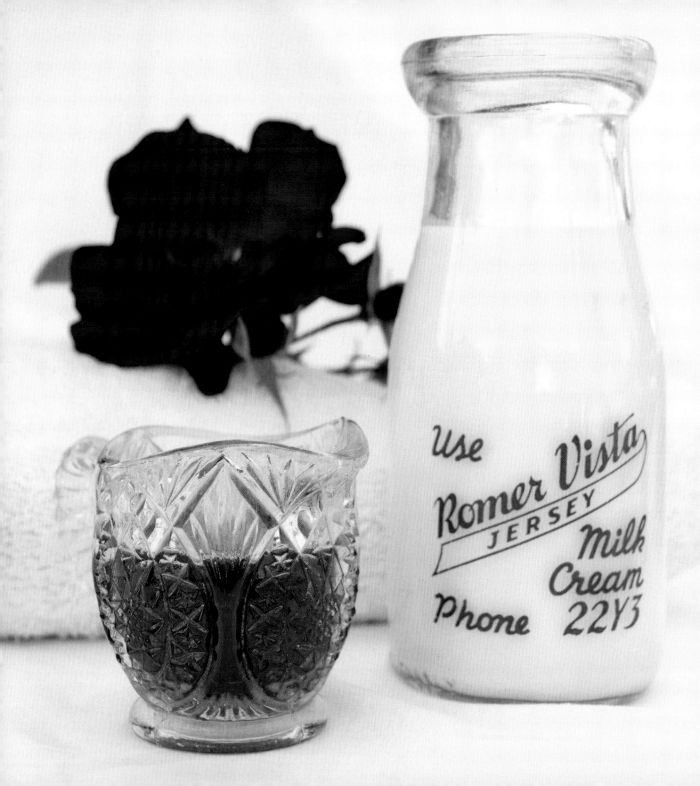

Coconut Rice
CONDITIONING EXFOLIANT

This luxurious, coconut-scented exfoliant for face and body is simply divine. For centuries, Asian cultures have used rice in skin care formulations to encourage clear, luminous, and porcelain skin. The rice gently exfoliates while the penetrating moisture from the coconut cream brings vitamins and minerals to the deeper dermal layers of your skin, helping to strengthen tissues while fighting fine lines, wrinkles, hyper-pigmentation, and dull, dry skin. Use this gorgeous head-to-toe skin treatment weekly to enhance your skin's natural luminosity.

YIELDS: *1 full body application*

¼ cup brown rice flour

¼ cup coconut shreds

Dash of ground nutmeg

⅔+ cup coconut cream
(full-fat coconut milk)

What you will need: medium-size mixing bowl, measuring cups, fork

❶ **To Make:** Place the brown rice flour, coconut shreds, and nutmeg in a medium-size mixing bowl and stir. Add the coconut cream and blend with a fork until you have a uniform consistency. Add more coconut cream, a little at a time as necessary to achieve a spreadable paste.

❷ **To Store:** This mask is best used fresh. Store any leftovers in a sealed container and use within 1–2 days.

❸ **To Use:** For best results, take a quick shower or use after a long soak in the tub. The warmth of the shower will open your pores and the moisture on your skin will provide a conduit for the mask to start working faster and more effectively. Towel dry and apply to skin in small, upward motions. Start with your body and finish with your face. Once you are covered from head to toe, massage the scrub in small circular motions, starting with the legs and arms, making your way up to the torso, ending at your heart. Then move to your face, avoiding the eye area. Massage your face with light pressure, using circular motions. Allow to set on your body for up to 30 minutes and up to 15 minutes on your face. To rinse, get in the shower and rinse well. For maximum benefit, do not use soap to wash off the residual oils. Towel dry and mist your face with Old-Fashioned Rosewater (see Chapter 7) to close the pores.

Ambrosia FACE AND BODY MASK

In Greek and Roman mythology, ambrosia is a food for the gods that is known to bestow immortality.
This luxurious home spa treatment may not help you live longer, but it will certainly give your skin
a more youthful glow! This highly moisturizing tropical treat exfoliates with natural fruit enzymes,
replenishes with vitamin C–packed fruits, and moisturizes with decadent coconut cream.
Enjoy this simply divine home spa experience to bring out the goddess in you.

YIELDS: *1 whole body mask*

½ cup pineapple

1 tablespoon fresh-squeezed orange juice

¼+ cup coconut cream

½ cup coconut flour

¼ cup granulated sugar

Zest of 1 orange

What you will need: blender, rubber spatula, mixing bowl, measuring cups, fork, tight-sealing storage container

1 **To Make:** Place the pineapple, orange juice, and coconut cream into the blender and mix on low until well blended. Place the creamed pineapple in the mixing bowl, using the rubber spatula to remove as much as possible. Add the coconut flour, sugar, and orange zest and stir with a fork until you have a uniform consistency. Add more coconut cream or sugar, a little at a time as necessary to achieve a spreadable paste.

2 **To Store:** This mask is best used fresh. Store any leftovers in a sealed container in the refrigerator and use within a day or 2.

3 **To Use:** Apply to clean, damp skin in small, upward motions. Start with your body and finish with your face. Once you are covered from head to toe, massage the scrub in small circular motions, starting with the legs and arms, making your way up to the torso, ending at your heart. Then move to your face, avoiding the eye area. Massage your face with light pressure, using circular motions. Allow to set on your body for up to 30 minutes and up to 15 minutes on your face. To rinse, get in the shower and rinse well. For maximum benefit, do not use soap to wash off the residual oils. Towel dry and mist your face with Old-Fashioned Rosewater (see Chapter 7) to close the pores. It is unlikely that you will need any additional moisturizer.

Vanilla Isle
PERFUME

Wearing perfume helps you feel luxurious and attractive, especially when you know it isn't made with harmful chemicals. Vanilla, an aphrodisiac, is combined with sultry ylang-ylang and flirty sweet orange in this soft and sexy scent. Anoint your pulse points with this gorgeous, all-natural, vanilla-y perfume with a tropical floral twist.

YIELDS: *2 ounces*

3 tablespoons Aromatic Vanilla Infusion (see Chapter 7)

1 tablespoon vanilla extract

8 drops patchouli essential oil

20 drops Australian sandalwood essential oil

24 drops ylang-ylang essential oil

44 drops sweet orange essential oil

1 tablespoon distilled water

What you will need: cutting board, knife, 2-ounce bottle with dropper top or spritz cap, small funnel

❶ **To Make:** Use a funnel to pour the Aromatic Vanilla Infusion and the vanilla extract into the bottle. Add the essential oils and fill up the bottle with distilled water. Cap it and shake well to blend.

❷ **To Store:** Label with expiration date of 2 years and store in a cool dark place out of direct sunlight.

❸ **To Use:** Shake well before each use. Apply to pulse points. Do not spray on lightly colored fabrics, as the vanilla may cause slight discoloration.

Blushing Bride
UBTAN EXFOLIANT

Ubtan is a luxurious traditional Indian pre-wedding spa treatment in which both the bride and groom are pampered with a series of aromatic facial and body masks coupled with massage for several days leading up to their wedding. This exotic home spa treatment is made from powdered herbs, flowers, and nuts combined with botanical oils and rosewater to create a nourishing, moisturizing, and exfoliating treat for your skin. Use this exotic aromatic beauty treatment from head to toe to gently slough off dull skin for super-soft skin with a healthy glow.

YIELDS: *1–2 full body masks*

¼ cup honey

¼ cup sweet almond oil or carrier oil of choice

¼–½ cup rosewater

1 cup Ayurvedic Facial Cleansing Grains (see Chapter 2)

What you will need: mixing bowl, fork, tight-sealing container

1 To Make: Place the honey, sweet almond oil, and ½ cup rosewater into the mixing bowl and beat together with a fork. Add in roughly ¼ cup of the cleansing grains and mix them together. Alternate adding more cleansing grains and rosewater a little at a time. Blend them in between additions until you've added all of the grains. Add enough rosewater to achieve a spreadable paste.

2 To Store: This is meant to be made just before use and applied fresh. Store any leftovers in a sealed container in the refrigerator and use up within a day or two.

3 To Use: For best results, take a quick shower or use after a long soak in the tub to soften your skin and remove surface dirt and toxins. The warmth of the shower will open your pores and the moisture on your skin will provide a conduit for the mask to start working faster and more effectively. Towel dry and apply to clean damp skin. Start with your

(continued on the following pages)

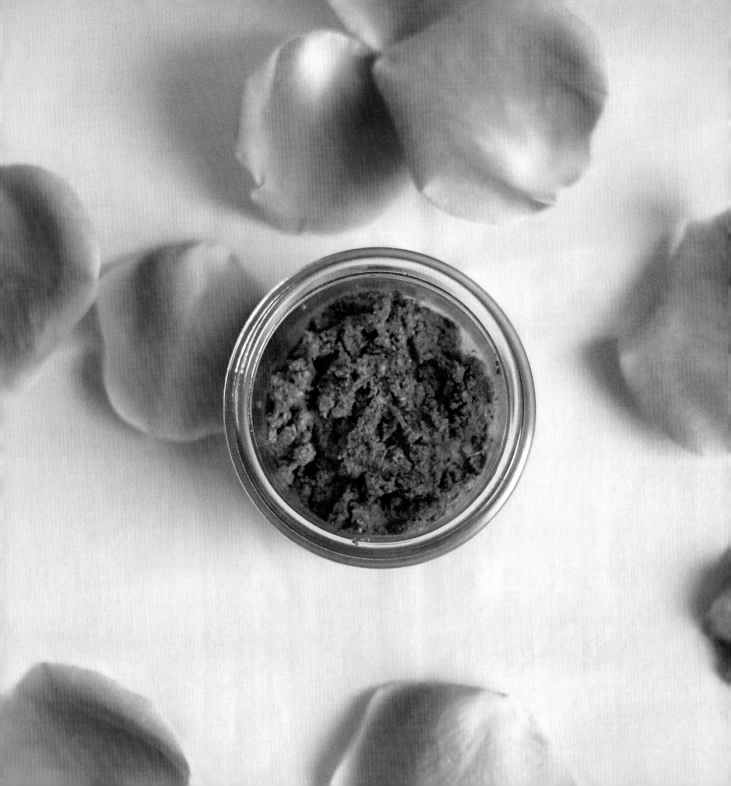

body, massaging the scrub in small circular motions as you go. Start with the legs and arms, making your way up to the torso, ending at your heart. Finish by applying a thin layer to your face, avoiding the eye area. Massage your face with light pressure, using circular motions. Once you are covered from head to toe, wrap yourself in plastic wrap, a clean sheet, or a towel and allow this to set for up to 30 minutes on your body and up to 15 minutes on your face. To rinse, get into a warm shower and rinse well. You may want to use a washcloth to help remove the mask from your face. Wet the cloth and apply to your face, leaving it to soak the mask from your skin, and then gently wipe off. Repeat a few times, rinsing in between. Use your fingertips and gently massage the wetted mask from your body. For maximum benefit, do not use soap to wash off the residual oils. Mist your face with Old-Fashioned Rosewater (see Chapter 7) to close the pores, and apply a facial moisturizer if desired.

SKIN CARE SECRETS

Traditionally, Ubtan would be followed by a luxurious bath and finished with a sensually scented moisturizer. Try the Coconut, Lime, and Rose Petals Bath from Chapter 6 and the Whipped Shea Body Butter from Chapter 5. Finish this luxury spa treatment by scenting your hair with the Jasmine Hair Finishing Oil from this chapter.

Detoxifying
SEAWEED BODY WRAP

Seaweed wraps are popular in high-end spas for their advanced body slimming, detoxification, and replenishing effects on the skin and the whole body. This Detoxifying Seaweed Body Wrap is formulated with antioxidant-rich green tea, magnesium-rich Epsom Salts, and kaolin clay, which work together to draw out the toxins, impurities, and excess water weight from your system while fortifying and re-mineralizing your cells. The coconut water increases hydration and the skin's ability to absorb nutrients, and the lavender essential oil brings a touch of relaxing aromatherapy, adding a fresh natural scent to temper the seaweed. This recipe will help alleviate cellulite, sluggish circulation, sore muscles, and dull or congested skin, and is beneficial for use on face and body for all skin types.

YIELDS: *1 full body application*

1 tablespoon Epsom salts

½-¾ cup coconut water

12 drops lavender essential oil

⅛ cup kelp powder

⅛ cup green tea powder

⅓ cup kaolin clay

What you will need: mixing bowl, measuring cups, fork, washcloth, plastic wrap, towels or blankets, 1 tight-sealing jar

❶ To Make: Dissolve the Epsom salts in the coconut water by placing in a mixing bowl and stirring gently with a fork. Add the lavender essential oil and stir. Add the kelp and green tea powders and stir gently. Lastly, add the kaolin clay and blend until you have a uniform consistency. If you need to adjust the texture, add more coconut water or kaolin clay a little at a time, as necessary to achieve an easily spreadable paste.

❷ To Store: This mask is best used fresh. You can mix the powders ahead of time and store them in a tight-sealing jar. Mix the coconut water with the powders fresh before each use. Store any leftovers in a sealed container in the refrigerator and use up within a day or 2.

③ To Use: Apply to clean damp skin in small, upward motions. Start with your body and finish with your face. Once you've covered your body, you can wrap yourself in plastic wrap to amplify the effect. This will be easier if you have someone help you, but it is possible to do it yourself. To get started, step on the end of the plastic and wrap up one leg at a time, wrap your torso, and then wrap one arm at a time. Wrap yourself in towels, a sheet, or blanket that you don't mind getting some of the mask on. Find a nice place to relax for at least 20 minutes, up to an hour for maximum benefit. Apply the mask to your face 15 minutes before you plan to wash off, avoiding the eye area. To remove, get in the shower and rinse well. Remove the mask from your face first and finish with your body. Do not scrub the mask off; rather, thoroughly saturate with water and gently wipe off with a soft cloth. Towel dry and apply your favorite moisturizer to your body. For your face, follow with toner and moisturizer.

SKIN CARE SECRETS

Remember to hydrate! With any type of detoxifying spa treatment, you can easily dehydrate while your body sweats out the toxins. Dehydrated cells are full of toxins, which can actually result in your body storing more water weight than it needs. Drink ample water on a regular basis, as it is helps your body process toxins by literally flushing them from your cells. Always drink plenty of fresh water for clear and beautiful skin.

Fizzy Mojito FOOT SPA

Treat yourself to this fresh and tingly home spa cocktail for your sore and tired feet! Astringent witch hazel helps relieve swelling, while the lime and grapefruit juices soften calluses. Mint refreshes and soothes, and the bubbly water re-mineralizes and relaxes. So get ready to relax and unwind while you enjoy this refreshing luxury spa pedicure!

YIELDS: *1 foot bath*

½ cup witch hazel

½ cup fresh-squeezed lime juice

½ cup fresh-squeezed grapefruit juice

1 lime, sliced into rings

1 quart sparkling mineral water

½ cup fresh mint leaves

½ cup Epsom salts

½ cup fine-grained sea salt

½ cup coconut cream
  (full-fat coconut milk)

What you will need: washtub, cutting board, wooden spoon, measuring cups, mixing bowl, fork Note: If you don't have a washtub, you can use a soup pot, shallow bowl, or plastic storage tub. As long as you can soak your feet inside without spilling, it should work!

1 **To Make:** Start with room temperature rather than refrigerated ingredients. Put the witch hazel, lime juice, grapefruit juice, and lime rings into the washtub with the mineral water. Muddle the mint leaves by crushing them with the back of a wooden spoon, coarsely chop them, put into the washtub, and give it a mix. In the mixing bowl, place the salts and coconut cream. Stir to blend to a uniform consistency. Bring the washtub and the bowl of scrub to the place where you will have your foot spa.

2 **To Store:** This recipe should be made fresh before each use.

3 **To Use:** Set up your foot spa area with anything you will want for a super comfy-cozy relaxing experience. Light a candle, gather a magazine or maybe an eye pillow, and enjoy a cup of tea. Play some relaxing music. Since the foot bath will not be warm, you may want a blanket, heating pad, and some pillows so you're sitting as comfortably as possible. Gather a towel to dry off after the foot bath. And you're ready to get started! Pour the mineral water into the washtub and stir. Settle in and soak your feet for 10–20 minutes. When you're ready, use the coconut cream and salt mix to scrub the built up dead skin and softened callouses off your toes and feet. Dry off with a towel. Rinse off your feet in the tub or shower if desired. Note: Get the most out of this foot spa treatment by trimming your toenails right before putting your feet to soak in the Fizzy Mojito Foot Spa. After the soak and scrub, use the tip of a nail file to scrape the softened buildup from under your nails.

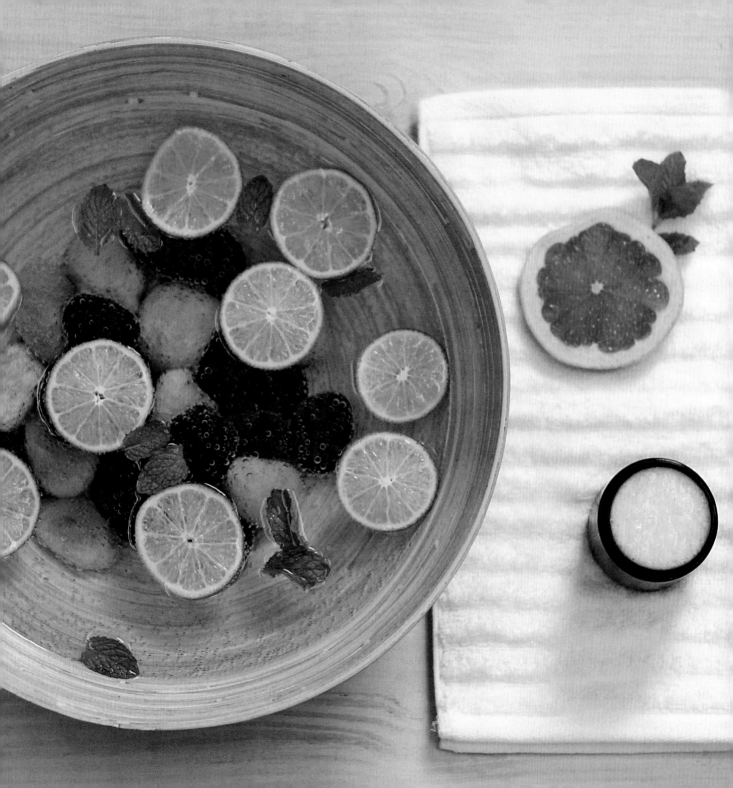

Soothing
SCALP AND HAIR TREATMENT

This botanical oil blend makes a deeply conditioning hair and scalp treatment for damaged hair and split ends as well as dry, flaky dandruff conditions. Enjoy a dreamy scalp massage to soothe uncomfortable scalp conditions, help unclog hair follicles, energize the scalp, oxygenate the roots, and stimulate hair growth while nourishing and deep conditioning your hair.

YIELDS: *8 ounces*

½ cup grapeseed oil

½ cup Rosemary-Infused Oil
(see Chapter 7) or jojoba oil

4 vitamin E capsules

10 drops rosemary essential oil

18 drops lemon essential oil

24 drops lavender essential oil

22 drops tea tree essential oil

What you will need: dark-colored 8-ounce bottle with a pump top (optional), comb or natural-bristled hairbrush, funnel

❶ To Make: Place the funnel over your bottle and add the grapeseed oil and Rosemary-Infused Oil. Pierce the vitamin E capsules and squeeze the liquid out into the bottle, discarding the gel caps. Add the essential oils, cap tightly, and shake to blend.

❷ To Store: Store in a cool, dry place out of direct sunlight and use up within 1 year.

❸ To Use: Ideally you want to start with brushed, tangle-free dry hair rather than wet or damp. If you have curly hair, you don't need to brush it out first. Apply generously to the scalp and then comb it through to the ends, applying more oil as necessary to reach full saturation. Massage the oil into your scalp with your fingertips for 10 minutes. Wrap your head in a towel and leave on for at least 30 minutes. The longer you are able to leave this conditioning oil on your hair and scalp, the better. Place a towel over your pillowcase and you can leave this on overnight. Wash and condition your hair as normal. It is suggested to clean your comb and brush after using them for this treatment.

HELPFUL HINTS

This treatment oil can also be used as a quick leave-in conditioning treatment or de-frizzer, or to help define ringlets in curly hair and bring out the texture in layered hair. Place a few drops of the oil onto your fingertips and run through the ends of your hair. You can apply this to wet or dry hair as needed.

Jasmine
HAIR FINISHING OIL

This gorgeously scented oil blend is formulated with nutritious sweet almond and olive oils that will effectively protect your hair, sealing moisture into the hair shaft and adding a luxe, healthy shine. This botanical treatment is nourishing, conditioning, and moisturizing for damaged hair and split ends—plus it smells absolutely divine!

YIELDS: *4 ounces*

¼ cup jojoba oil

¼ cup extra-virgin olive oil

2 vitamin E capsules

20 drops sweet orange essential oil

12 drops rose geranium essential oil

16 drops patchouli or Australian sandalwood essential oil

28 drops Jasmine Absolute oil

What you will need: dark-colored 4-ounce bottle with a pump top (optional), funnel, pint-sized container

1 **To Make:** Place the funnel over your pint-size container and add the jojoba oil and olive oil. Pierce the vitamin E capsules and squeeze the liquid out into the bottle, discarding the gel caps. Add the essential oils and Jasmine Absolute, cap tightly, and shake to blend.

2 **To Store:** Store in a cool, dry place out of direct sunlight and use up within a year.

3 **To Use:** Use this luxuriously scented oil as a quick leave-in conditioning treatment or de-frizzer, or to help define ringlets and texturize layered hair. Place a few drops of the oil onto your fingertips and run through the ends of your hair. Tousle the waves, twisting the ends of your hair to texturize. Apply to wet, damp, or dry hair as needed.

Sunrise
SPA WATER

Greet the day with a toast to your health and happiness! This sunny beverage makes a gorgeous addition to a home spa party, as the juices layer in the glass like a beautiful sunrise. High in vitamin C and antioxidants, the citrus fruit aids digestion and liver cleansing, and the pomegranate juice is packed with beneficial vitamins and antioxidants that fight free radicals. Pomegranate is also anti-inflammatory and heart-healthy and has been shown to protect the system from certain cancers.

YIELDS: *about 8 cups*

4 cups water

1 orange, sliced thin

1 Meyer lemon, sliced thin

2 tablespoons agave or honey, optional

3 cups unsweetened pomegranate juice (or cranberry or cherry Juice)

16–24 ice cubes, optional

What you will need: knife, cutting board, half-gallon pitcher, long-handled spoon, strainer

1. **To Make:** Begin the preparation the night before you plan to serve. Mix the water with citrus fruit slices and agave, if desired, in a pitcher. Refrigerate overnight, allowing the flavors to infuse the water.

2. **To Store:** Store in the fridge for up to 4 days.

3. **To Use:** For an extra special layered juice "sunrise" presentation, place 2–3 ice cubes in a clear glass. Add ½ cup pomegranate juice. Slowly fill glasses the rest of the way with the strained citrus water. Garnish with a slice of sunshine and a citrus slice and serve. Or, add the pomegranate juice to the pitcher and stir. Serve over ice if desired.

SKIN CARE SECRETS

For truly healthy skin, you must eat well and hydrate, hydrate, hydrate! Every cell in your body is reliant on water for proper function, and a hydrated body is a healthy body is a beautiful body.

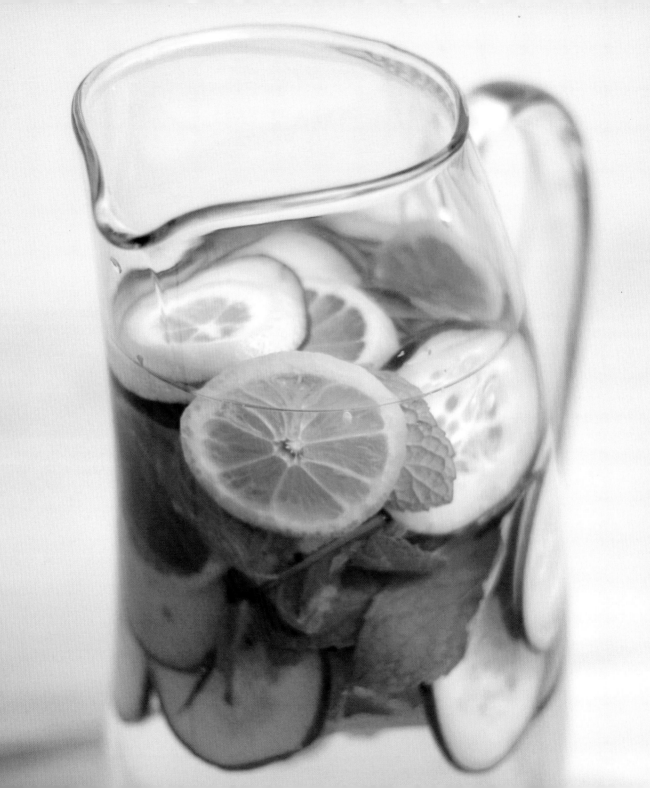

Cucumber
DE-PUFFER SPA WATER

Get rid of extra water weight while staying hydrated with this deliciously quenching spa water. Cucumber and lemon are natural diuretics that aid digestion and appetite control. The ginger and spearmint help relieve bloating and will also benefit the digestive system. This delicious, refreshing, and detoxifying drink is beneficial for weight loss and for relieving PMS symptoms.

YIELDS: *8 cups*

8 cups spring water

5 thin slices of ginger, peeled

1 medium cucumber, sliced thin

1 medium lemon, sliced thin

12 spearmint leaves

ice, optional

cucumber, optional

What you will need: knife, cutting board, half-gallon pitcher, strainer, long-handled spoon

1 **To Make:** Mix all the ingredients together in a large pitcher. Refrigerate for several hours or overnight to allow the flavors to infuse the water. Strain and serve over ice, if desired. Garnish with a slice of cucumber or lemon.

2 **To Store:** Keep refrigerated and drink within 4 days.

3 **To Use:** You can drink this spa water all day long! Drink this for up to four days in a row and you will start feeling great. The extra fluids and diuretics are flushing out the toxins while you are also flooding your system with vitamin C, antioxidants, and digestive aids. You are cleaning out your cells and staying hydrated, which will show in the radiance, tone, and texture of your skin.

SKIN CARE SECRETS

The ingredient combinations in these spa waters are specifically formulated to support healthy skin texture and appearance while providing a good dose of anti-aging vitamin C. Additional benefits include appetite control, immune defense, heartburn prevention, blood sugar regulation, and weight management. What a fun and delicious way to care for your skin!

Strawberry
SUPER C SIPPER

Delicious strawberries and kiwis, which are both superfoods, have anti-aging properties and are full of vitamin C, antioxidants, and phytonutrients. Diets high in vitamin C promote healthier skin, and this spa water will leave yours beaming with vitality. With a spa water that tastes this good, you won't even need to be reminded to drink up and drink often!

YIELDS: *8 cups*

7 cups spring water

1 pint strawberries, trimmed and halved

1 small kiwi, sliced into thin rounds

1 tablespoon fresh lemon juice

Strawberry Basil Ice Cubes, optional
(see sidebar)

What you will need: knife, cutting board, half-gallon pitcher, long-handled spoon

❶ **To Make:** Mix all ingredients together in a large pitcher. Refrigerate for at least 2 hours.

❷ **To Store:** Store in the fridge for up to 4 days.

❸ **To Use:** Put some ice in your glass, fill it up with the Strawberry Super C Sipper, and enjoy. This is so good for you!

SKIN CARE SECRETS

To make Strawberry and Basil Ice Cubes, mash or purée strawberries with enough water to make them slushy. Fill an ice cube tray with the mixture. Place a fresh basil leaf in each cube and freeze. Why basil? It's a flavorful herb that packs a powerful punch when it comes to advancing overall health and well-being. Amazing—and delicious!

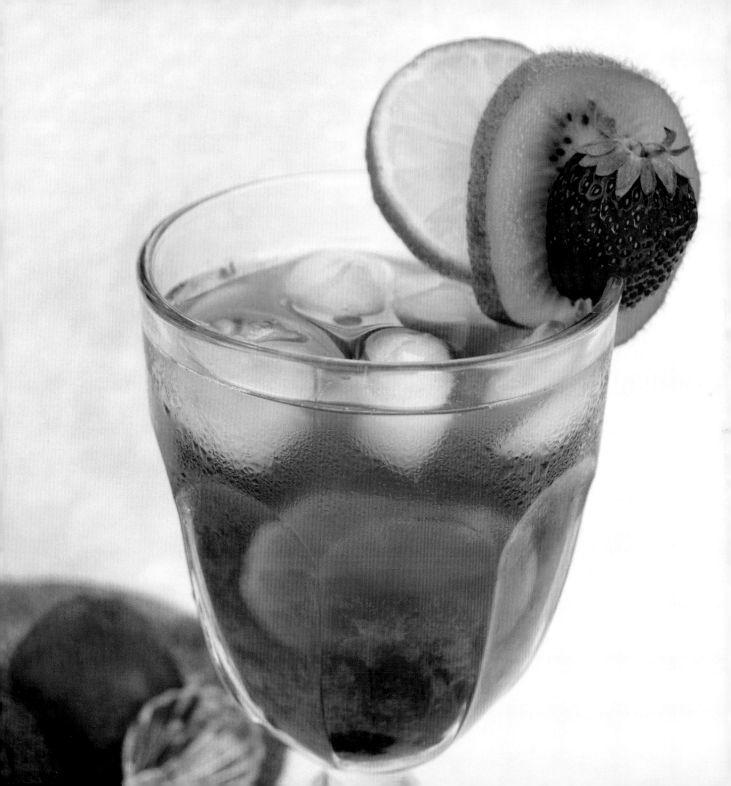

Quick Coconut
CANTALOUPE COOLER

The nutritional diversity of cantaloupe is perhaps its most overlooked health benefit! High in vitamins C, A, K, and a host of B's as well as potassium, magnesium, and fiber, this Quick Coconut Cantaloupe Cooler gives you a clear, hydrated complexion and shiny hair. With a healthy, delicious beverage that gives you an overall feeling of wellness, how can you go wrong?

YIELDS: *8 cups*

½ ripe cantaloupe, cut into small pieces

3 cups chilled water

2 cups chilled coconut water (or substitute aloe water)

1 lime, sliced into thin rounds

Ice

Mint for garnish

What you will need: cutting board, knife, food processor or blender (optional), juice pitcher

1 **To Make:** Divide your cut cantaloupe in half. Purée half of it in a food processor or blender, or smash it up with a fork. Add some of the water to the blender if necessary to achieve the purée. Put the cantaloupe purée into the pitcher. Mix in the water, coconut water, lime, and the rest of the cubed cantaloupe, and ice.

2 **To Store:** Store in the fridge and drink within 4 days.

3 **To Use:** Stir and serve immediately over ice. Garnish with a sprig of mint.

Rosy Green Tea
SPA WATER

Green tea and rose hips are rich in vitamins and antioxidants, bioflavonoids, and alkaloids.
This calming brew promotes healthy skin and hair and has detoxifying properties.
Enjoy this delicious and refreshing immune-boosting elixir
with the subtle scent of roses.

YIELDS: *8 cups*

2 roses in full bloom

8 cups spring water

2 tablespoons green tea

¼ cup dried rose hips

1 teaspoon rosewater, optional

Ice, optional

What you will need: large saucepan, strainer, half-gallon pitcher, wooden spoon

❶ **To Make:** Choose robustly blooming roses to pluck the petals from for this recipe. Remove the petals from one rose directly after cutting from the plant to preserve the highest nutrient value and reserve. Place the other in a vase to brighten your workspace. Bring the water to boiling in a saucepan and remove from heat. Let the water cool a minute and add the green tea and rose hips to the pan, stirring to saturate. Steep for 3–5 minutes and strain the liquid into a pitcher. Let cool for 20 minutes then add the rosewater and the petals from one rose and stir. Serve warm or refrigerate 30 minutes and serve chilled over ice, if desired.

❷ **To Store:** Store in the fridge and drink within 4 days.

❸ **To Use:** Drink up to 3 glasses a day. Serve over ice if desired.

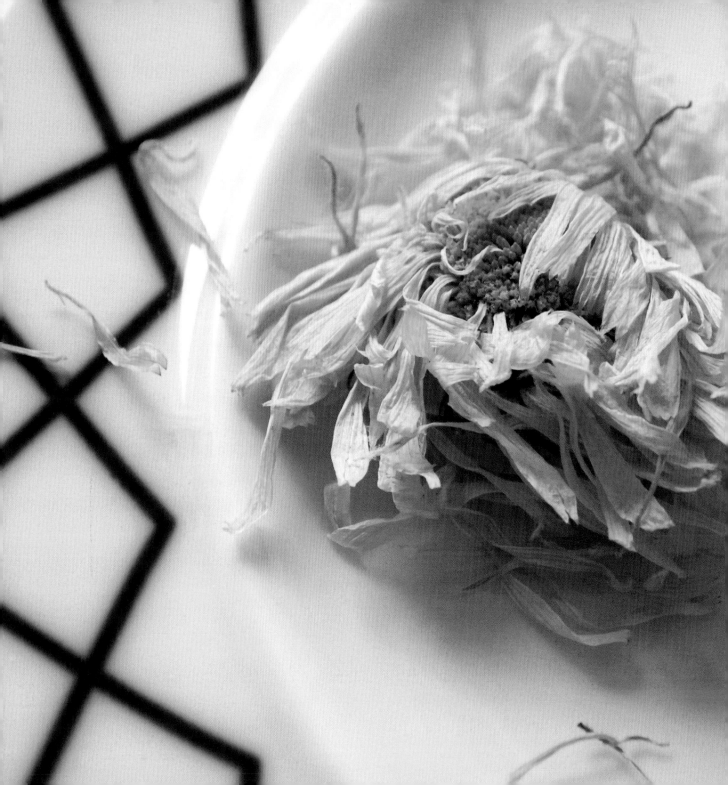

CHAPTER 9

SUN CARE

The sun's rays are getting stronger every year, and overexposure to UVA and UVB ultraviolet rays is one of the leading causes of premature aging, wrinkling, age spots, and, of course, skin cancer. Sun exposure is often accompanied with wind and water, an extremely drying combination to the skin. We all know it's best to not overdo it when it comes to the sun, so before you head out, protect your skin by slathering up with the Sun Protection Lotion Stick, wear a hat, and stay out of the sun between 11 A.M. and 2 P.M., when its rays are the strongest.

While a suntan may look like a healthy glow, it is your body's primary defense mechanism against the sun. The best thing you can do for overexposed and sun-damaged skin is to keep it moisturized and feed it with high levels of antioxidants both in the foods you eat and the skin care products you choose.

Help your skin combat the drying effects of the sun by moisturizing before and after sun exposure with the Calming Antioxidant Skin Quencher. If you overdo it, use the healing skin care products in this chapter for gentle relief like the Soothe-My-Sunburn Bath and the Cucumber Rose Sunburn Relief. Get that carefree, endless summer style any time of year by using the Beachy Babe Hair Spray for naturally texturized, super-cute surfer-girl waves to complement your healthy, glowing skin.

Sun-Kissed
PRE-TANNING BODY SCRUB

Exfoliate at least once per week to remove built-up dead skin cells. Healthy, regularly moisturized and exfoliated skin will allow you to tan more evenly. Sun exposure is much healthier when you use the appropriate precautions. Remember your hat and sunscreen and stay out of the sun during the middle of the day, when its rays are the strongest.

YIELDS: *12 ounces*

1 cup fine-grained sea salt

½ cup grapeseed oil

16 drops sweet orange essential oil

14 drops lavender essential oil

10 drops tea tree essential oil

What you will need: measuring cup, mixing bowl, fork, 12-ounce jar

1 **To Make:** Place salt into a mixing bowl. Add the grapeseed oil and essential oils. Stir until you have a uniform consistency and it's ready to use!

2 **To Store:** To preserve the freshness of this natural scrub, do not get water into the jar. Store this scrub a sealed jar in a cool dark place, out of direct sunlight. Label with expiration date of 1 year.

3 **To Use:** Use in place of a soap or body wash in your shower or bath. Apply to your skin in small, upward, circular motions. Massage the scrub in small circular motions, starting with the legs and arms, making your way up to the torso, ending at your heart. Rinse well.

SKIN CARE SECRETS

This scrub is designed to leave oils on your skin. For maximum benefit, do not use soap to wash off the residual oils. Towel off and the nutrients in the botanical oils will greatly benefit your skin, soaking in after a few minutes. You will not likely need any additional moisturizer. Avoid any open wounds and use caution, as the shower floor may become slippery. Not recommended for use on sunburned skin or open wounds.

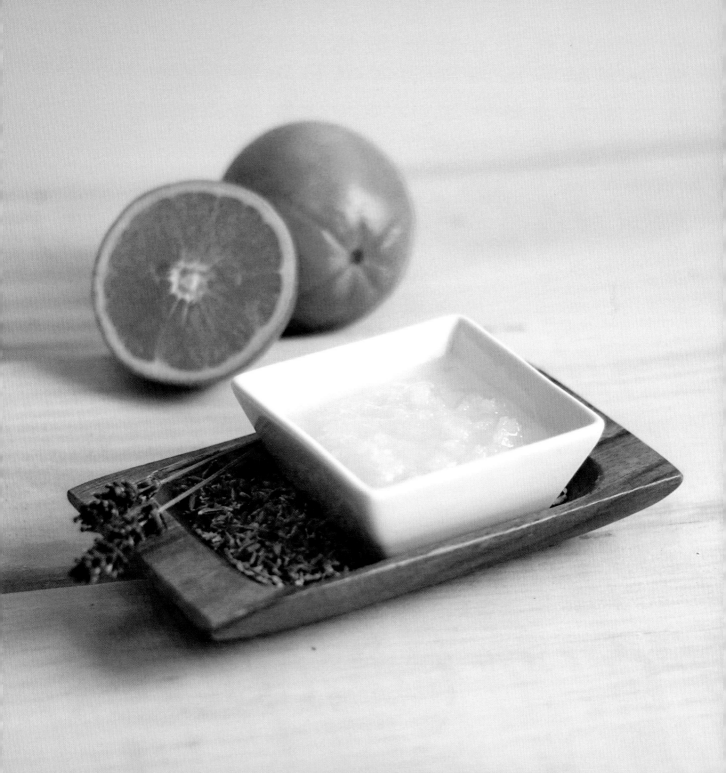

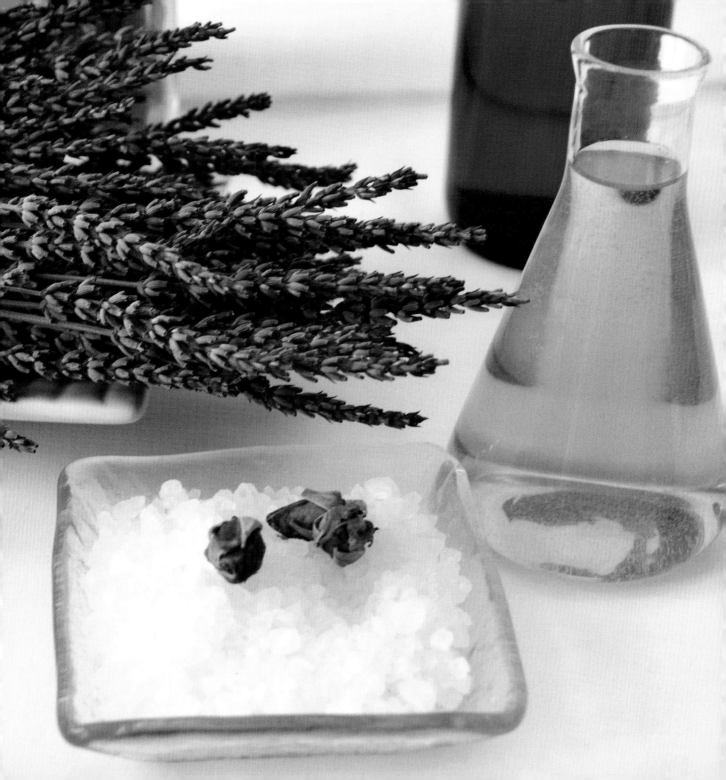

Yogurt Lavender Comfort
BODY MASK AND BATH

Have fun slathering yourself from head to toe with this silky, cooling, moisturizing yogurt mask. The natural emollients and lactic acid in yogurt provide a safe and gentle, nonabrasive moisturizing exfoliation. Be sure to use full-fat yogurt, as your sun-kissed skin needs the extra moisture.

YIELDS: *makes a single use*

1–2 cups full-fat plain yogurt, chilled

1 tablespoon baking soda

4 drops lavender essential oil

¼ cup dried lavender buds

2 or more cucumber slices, optional

What you will need: measuring cups, cheesecloth, string, bowl, fork

1 To Make: Run a lukewarm bath, not hot. The cooler, the better, but it should be warm enough to sit in for at least 10 minutes. Place the yogurt and baking soda in a bowl and mix well with a fork. Stir in the essential oil. Apply the cool yogurt mixture to your skin from head to toe. Place the lavender buds inside of the cheesecloth to form a loose sachet, leaving room for the water to flow through and the buds to plump in the bath water. Tie closed with a string and put it into the tub.

2 To Store: Make fresh for each use.

3 To Use: When the tub is full, get in and let the relaxation begin. The yogurt mask will dissolve off of your body and mingle with the lavender, creating a milky, moisturizing, relaxing elixir for mind, body, and spirit. Use the lavender sachet as a soothing wash bag by filling with water and squeezing out over your sore, sunburned skin. Use it as a spot treatment and compress. Place the cucumber slices over your eyes or directly on sunburned areas as a cooling anti-inflammatory treatment. Leave the yogurt on your face for up to 15 minutes. Drain the tub and rinse off with a quick shower. Gently towel dry and generously moisturize while your skin is still damp.

Avo-Oat After-Sun
FACE AND BODY MASK

Exposure to the sun, wind, salt, and sand often creates dry, flaky skin, which can be remedied with this Avo-Oat After-Sun Face and Body Mask. Nutrient-rich emollient avocados work to heal sun-damaged and weather-worn skin and help reduce the appearance of age spots. Keep your skin looking beautiful after a day in the sunshine with this soothing, replenishing all-over body mask that is packed with therapeutic ingredients to gently exfoliate while helping to moisturize, repair, and condition sun-kissed skin.

YIELDS: *1 full body treatment*

Flesh of 2 ripe avocados

2 teaspoons fresh lemon juice

2 tablespoons extra-virgin olive oil

1 cup cooked oatmeal

2 cups fine granulated sugar

What you will need: medium-size mixing bowl, large fork, measuring cups and spoons, tight-sealing container

❶ **To Make:** Mash the flesh of the avocados with a large fork. Stir in the lemon juice and olive oil. Stir in the oatmeal. Next, add the sugar and mix into an even paste. The texture should be easily spreadable and not too chunky. Add more olive oil if it's too thick or more sugar if it's too thin, 1 teaspoon at a time to find the perfect consistency.

❷ **To Store:** Store in tightly sealed container in the refrigerator for up to 3 days. Reduce the airspace in the storage container to help prevent oxidation.

❸ **To Use:** This recipe is appropriate for sun-kissed, not sunburned, skin. If you have a sunburn, choose another recipe from this chapter such as the Soothe-My-Sunburn Bath. Apply a thick layer to clean damp skin. Start with the body and finish with the face, avoiding eye area. Leave on 10–30 minutes. You can wrap yourself in plastic wrap, a clean sheet, and/or sit on a towel or lay in the tub. To remove, moisten your skin and massage the mask off in small circular motions, starting with the legs and arms, making your way up to the torso, ending at your heart.

Calming Antioxidant
SKIN QUENCHER

This luxuriously calming, healing moisturizer is rich in regenerative antioxidants that counteract the damaging effects of the sun's rays. This botanical infusion is steeped with the advanced healing powers of green tea and soothing comfrey combined with lavender to nurture you in mind, body, and spirit.

YIELDS: *4 ounces*

¼ cup Green Tea–Infused Oil (see Chapter 7)

¼ cup Fresh Comfrey Oil (see Chapter 7)

3 vitamin E capsules

20 drops lavender essential oil

What you will need: funnel, dark-colored 4-ounce bottle and cap

1 **To Make:** Use a funnel to pour the Green Tea–Infused Oil and Fresh Comfrey Oil into a 4-ounce bottle. Pierce the vitamin E capsules and squeeze the liquid out into the bottle, discarding the gel caps. Add lavender essential oil. Place cap on tightly and shake well to blend.

2 **To Store:** Store in a cool dry place out of direct sunlight. Label with expiration date of 2 years.

3 **To Use:** Body oils are best applied right after bathing, while the skin is still damp. The oils work to seal in the moisture on your skin. And the moisture on your skin works to deliver the active botanicals deeper into the dermal layers of your skin.

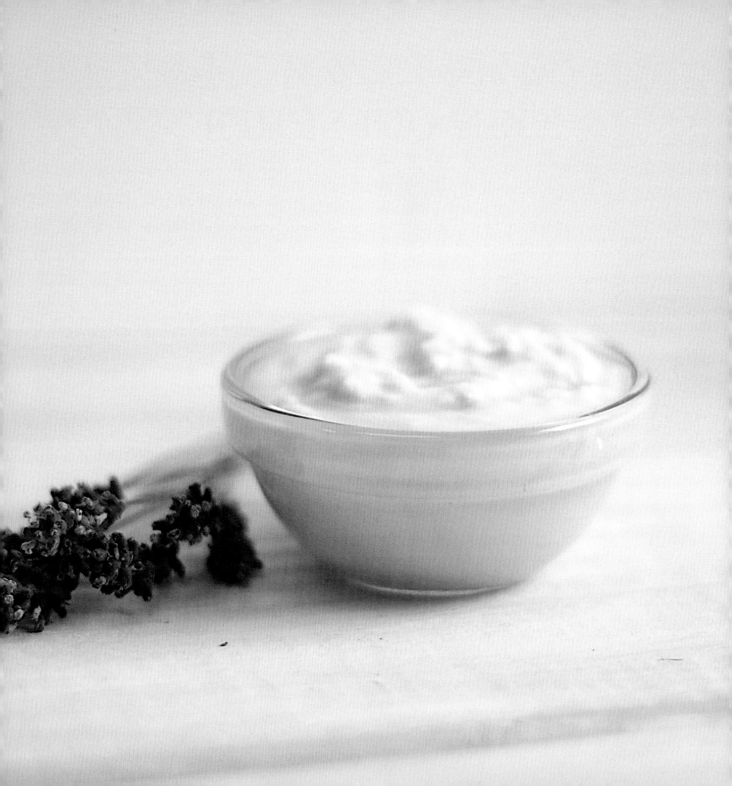

Cooling
ANTI-ITCH PASTE

Topical application of this simple apple cider vinegar and baking soda paste can help ease sunburn pain, itching, and inflammation. How? Well, apple cider vinegar contains acetic acid, which is one of the components of pain relief medications such as aspirin. Smear on this Cooling Anti-Itch Paste for some all-natural relief to help you feel better fast.

YIELDS: *1 cup*

½ cup apple cider vinegar

½ cup baking soda

6 drops lavender essential oil, optional

What you will need: bowl, spoon, tight-sealing storage container

❶ **To Make:** Place all ingredients in a bowl and mix to form a thick paste.

❷ **To Store:** Store in the refrigerator in a sealed container for up to 2 weeks. Stir well before each use.

❸ **To Use:** Apply to sunburned or itchy spots. Leave on for as long as you like. To remove, rinse or shower off. To avoid irritating your skin, do not rub or scrub off. If you are really suffering, consider applying before bed. Allow to dry completely before getting into bed. Not recommended to leave on your face overnight.

Soothe-My-Sunburn BATH

Baking soda creates an alkalized environment that is soothing to the skin. It has antiseptic properties, can help with the itch, and works as an exfoliant. Adding baking soda to this simple bath can ease sunburn pain, itching, and inflammation and get you back on the beach in no time!

YIELDS: *2–3 baths*

1 cup baking soda

1 cup raw oatmeal

2 cups dried comfrey leaves

Apple cider vinegar, 2 cups per bath

What You Will Need: measuring cups, rubber gloves, mixing bowl, cheesecloth, string, tight-sealing storage container

1. **To Make:** Place the baking soda, oatmeal, and comfrey leaves in the mixing bowl. Put on the rubber gloves and blend the ingredients together with your hands, crushing the comfrey leaves and oats into the baking soda, making a uniform mixture. Run a lukewarm bath, not hot. The cooler the better, but it should be warm enough to sit in for at least 10 minutes. Place 1 cup of the bath mix inside of the cheesecloth and tie closed to form a loose sachet. Leave room in the sachet for the water to flow through and the oats to plump in the bath water. Tie closed with a rubber band or string and put it into the tub. When the tub is full, add 2 cups of apple cider vinegar and swish to blend.

2. **To Store:** Store in a tightly sealed container.

3. **To Use:** Get in the tub and let the relaxation begin. Use the oatmeal sachet as a soothing wash bag by filling with water and squeezing out over your sore, sunburned skin. Use it as a spot treatment and compress. Place cucumber slices over your eyes or sunburned areas as a cooling anti-inflammatory treatment. Drain the tub and rinse off with a quick shower. Gently towel dry and generously moisturize while your skin is still damp.

SKIN CARE SECRETS

Special instructions for a sunburn bath: Use warm to cool water to soothe the burn. Don't use soap, bubble bath, or bath salts, as they can be drying to sunburned skin. Also, don't use a washcloth, brush, or any sort of intense exfoliant until your skin is healing. You don't want to soak too long and dry out your skin, so limit the bath to 10–15 minutes. Sunburns are very drying to your skin, so drink lots of water to moisturize from the inside out. Be sure to apply a moisturizer as soon as you get out of the tub, providing your skin a protective moisture barrier, helping to speed healing and prevent peeling.

Healing Sunburn
SPRAY AND COMPRESS

There is nothing like a cool mist of this Healing Sunburn Spray and Compress to soothe your tender overexposed skin. The green tea used in this recipe contains tannic acid, theobromine, and polyphenols— all of which are soothing and healing to sunburned skin. In addition, yerba mate is a South American super-antioxidant that helps speed tissue repair. With the addition of cooling peppermint and the skin healers chamomile and aloe vera, this concoction is sure to soothe the sting of a sunburn!

YIELDS: *1 quart*

4 cups filtered or spring water

¼ cup fresh peppermint leaves

¼ cup fresh chamomile flowers

1 tablespoon loose leaf yerba mate

1 tablespoon green tea leaves

½ cup aloe vera juice

10 drops peppermint essential oil

What you will need: kettle, large saucepan, spoon, strainer, quart jar, spray bottle

1 **To Make:** Boil 4 cups of water in the saucepan. Remove from heat and add the herbs and tea, stirring with a spoon to moisten thoroughly. Let the infusion steep for 15–20 minutes. Strain the herbs from the brew and pour into the jar. Place in the fridge and cool completely, 15–20 minutes. Once the brew has cooled, add the aloe vera and essential oil. Seal the lid tightly and shake well to blend.

2 **To Store:** Pour some of the mixture into a spray bottle. Reserve the remainder in the jar. Store in the refrigerator for up to 2 weeks.

3 **To Use:** Shake before use. Spray affected areas as desired. Soak a soft cloth and apply as a compress for 10–15 minutes to affected areas.

HELPFUL HINTS

If you do not have access to fresh peppermint, chamomile, loose leaf yerba mate, or loose leaf green tea, substitute tea bags: 1 peppermint, 1 chamomile, 1 yerba mate, 1 green tea. Make sure the tea bags contain only the pure herb, without any flavorings or additional blended herbs.

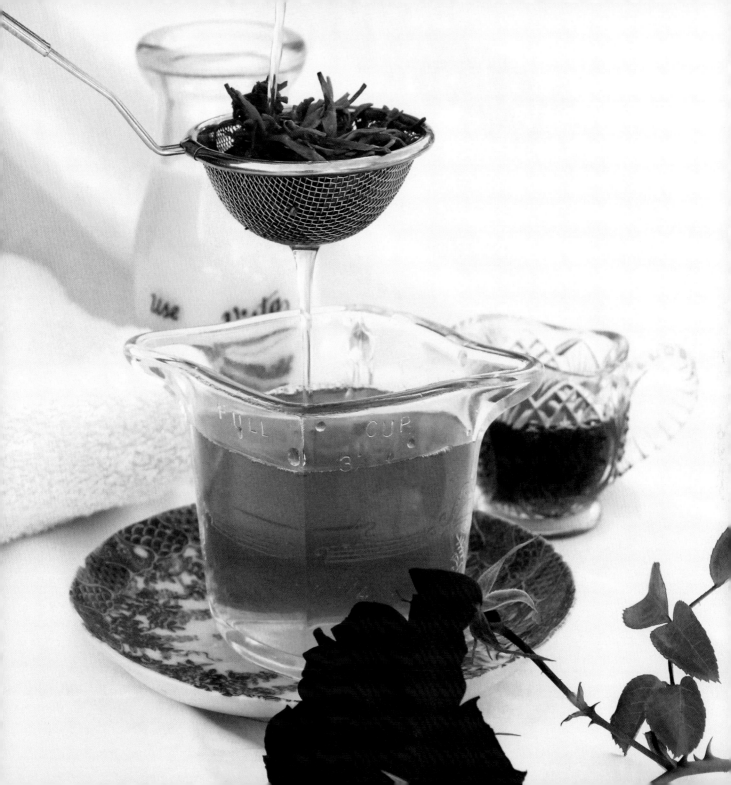

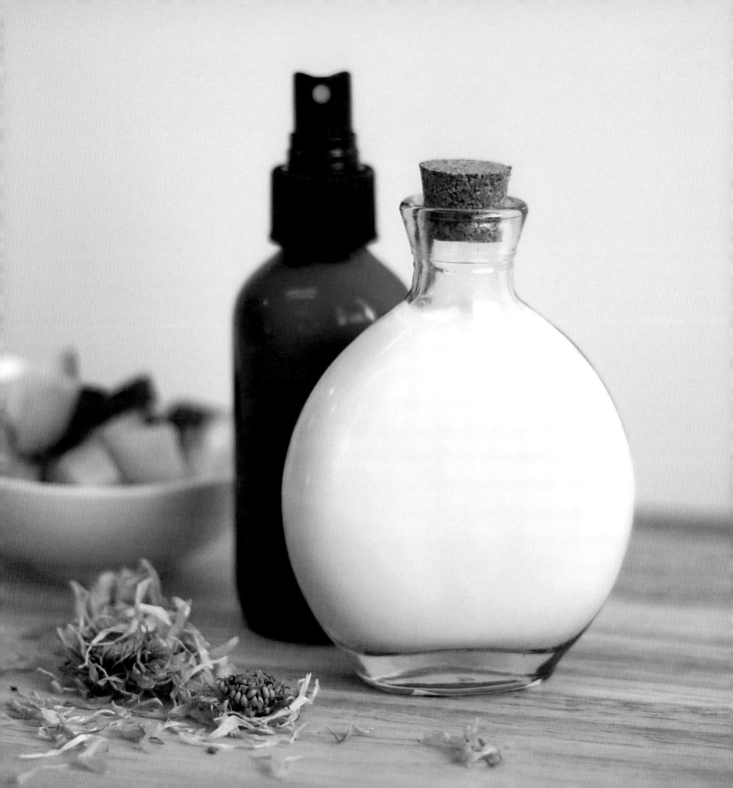

Cucumber Rose
SUNBURN RELIEF

You will want to have this cooling, fragrant, milky lotion on hand after a long day in the sun. Store this concoction in the fridge and mist this soothing, moisturizing blend on a sunburn for instant relief. The aloe vera and cucumber provide instant anti-inflammatory relief, while the rose and coconut milk offer skin-saving healing moisture to overexposed skin.

YIELDS: *approximately 1 cup*

1 medium-size cucumber, chopped

¼ cup coconut milk

¼ cup Old-Fashioned Rosewater (see Chapter 7)

¼ cup aloe vera juice

What you will need: strainer or cheesecloth, 8-ounce jar with lid, spray bottle

1 **To Make:** Put the chopped cucumber inside a strainer or piece of cheesecloth and squeeze out juice. Pour the cucumber juice into a jar. Add coconut milk, rosewater, and aloe vera. Close the lid tightly and shake well to blend.

2 **To Store:** Pour some of the mixture into a spray bottle. Reserve the remainder in the jar. Store in the refrigerator for up to 1 week.

3 **To Use:** Shake well before use. Spray affected areas as desired. Soak a soft cloth and apply as a compress for 10–15 minutes to affected areas.

Sun Protection
LOTION STICK

Certain plants have amazing sun protection properties: shea butter has an SPF of around 7, coconut oil's SPF is around 4, and red raspberry seed oil has an SPF ranging between 28 and 50. This recipe combines these amazing sun-blocking botanicals with zinc, a mineral that physically blocks the sun by scattering UVA and UVB radiation, to create nourishing and effective natural sun protection. The butter-like consistency of this recipe adds to its effectiveness by creating natural sweat and water resistance, and the peppermint helps keep you cool. Enjoy!

YIELDS: *4 two-ounce tubes*

2 tablespoons beeswax pastilles

¼ cup shea butter

¼ cup coconut oil (virgin or unscented or green tea–infused (see Chapter 7))

¼ cup red raspberry seed oil

20 drops peppermint essential oil

4 vitamin E capsules

2 tablespoons zinc oxide powder

What you will need: double boiler, measuring cups, rubber spatula, push-up tubes for 8-ounce recipe (four 2-ounce tubes)

1 **To Make:** Start the double boiler on medium heat. Once it reaches a boil, reduce heat to simmer. Place the beeswax, shea butter, and coconut oil in the top of the double boiler and cover. Simmer until melted, stirring occasionally. To preserve the beneficial botanicals, do not overheat. Remove from heat, take the top pan off the double boiler, and let cool 5–10 minutes. Add the raspberry seed oil and essential oil. Pierce the vitamin E capsules and squeeze the liquid out into the bottle, discarding the gel caps. Add the zinc, being mindful not to breathe the powder. Carefully stir in the zinc powder, blending to a uniform mixture.

2 This last stage is a delicate balance of temperature. You don't want to pour it so hot that the zinc settles to the bottom of your tubes, but you need it to be warm enough to pour. Let cool until it just barely begins to thicken, another 5 minutes or so. Stir again to evenly disperse the zinc and pour into your tubes, scraping any of the hardened cooled mixture off the sides and back into the melted oils. If the mixture hardens too much before you can pour it, gently melt it again in the double boiler. Pour into the lotion tubes and let stand undisturbed for 4 hours or overnight.

❸ **To Store:** Store in a cool dry place out of direct sunlight. Use up within a year.

❹ **To Use:** Apply to skin at least 20 minutes before sun exposure. Reapply after swimming and exercise.

SKIN CARE SECRETS

You can make this recipe into lotion bars instead of the push-up tubes. Follow the directions given. Pour the melted butter into an ice cube tray, silicone mold, or a loaf pan lined with wax paper. Let stand at least 4 hours before moving. You can store the lotion bars in metal tins, wrapped in foil, or in a glass jar.

Beachy Babe
HAIR SPRAY

Love the perfectly messy free-spirited look of your hair after a day at the beach? This easy recipe will keep your locks surfer-sexy year round. Use extra-virgin coconut oil to get the natural coconut scent and the excellent conditioning properties that counteracts the salt and vodka.

YIELDS: *10 ounces*

1 cup distilled water

1½ tablespoons sea salt

1 teaspoon extra-virgin coconut oil

1 teaspoon aloe vera juice

1 tablespoon 80 proof vodka

OPTIONAL ADD-INS

Brew 1 chamomile tea bag in the water for lightening effects

Brown hair: Brew 1 black tea bag in the water

Add 1 teaspoon hair gel, unscented or with a scent complementary to the natural coconut scent. This helps to hold the waves in your hair longer.

What you will need: kettle, measuring cups and spoons, 10-ounce spray bottle, funnel

1 **To Make:** Bring the water to almost boiling and remove from heat. If brewing the optional chamomile or black tea, steep 5 minutes and discard the tea bags. Put the sea salt, coconut oil, and hair gel (optional) into the bottle. Use a funnel to carefully transfer the hot water (or brewed tea) into your spray bottle. Shake well to dissolve the ingredients. Let cool completely. Now add the aloe vera juice and vodka. Shake well and you're good to go!

2 **To Store:** The Beachy Babe Hair Spray is good for up to 3 months, 4 months if stored in the refrigerator. Placing in the refrigerator will cause the coconut oil to harden, however. If this occurs, just warm it back up by placing in hot water for a few minutes, shake well, and enjoy! Remember to label with contents and expiration date.

3 **To Use:** Shake well before each use, as the ingredients will separate. Spray generously onto damp or dry hair. Scrunch and twist into beachy waves. This works best if you air-dry. If you must blow dry, tousle on low with the hair dryer in short bursts, continually scrunching, making beachy-fabulous waves.

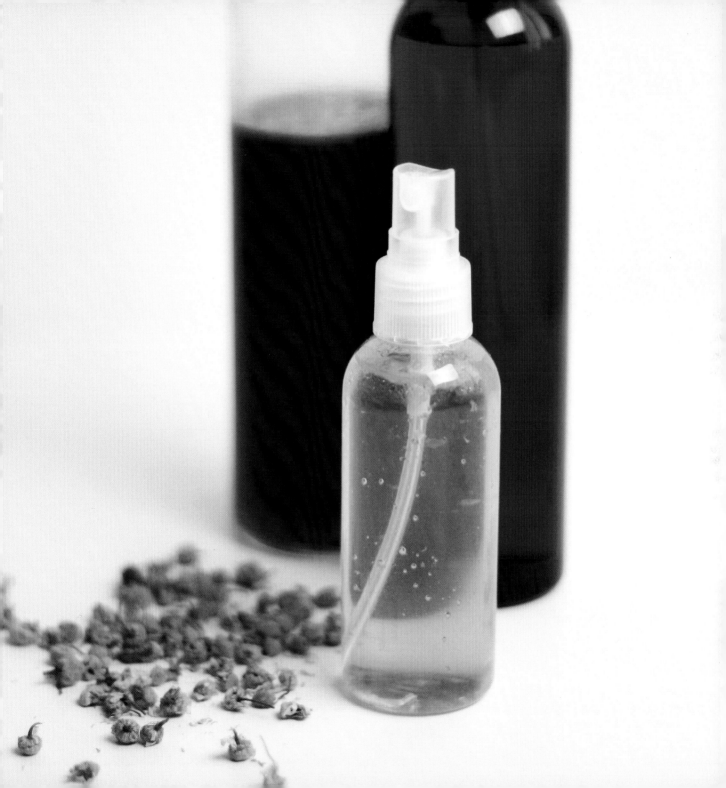

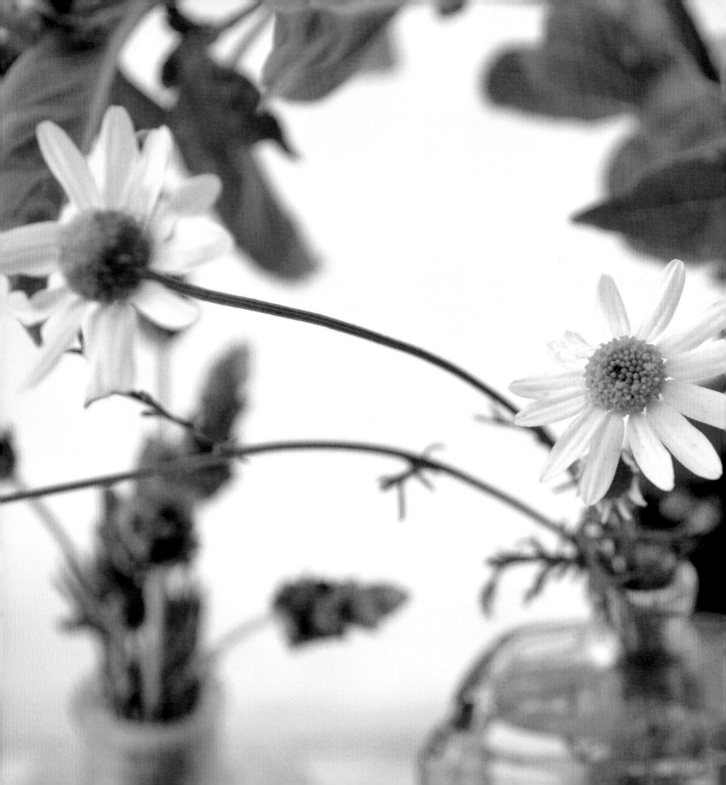

ESSENTIAL OIL BLENDS

The following Essential Oil Blends were created to scent an eight-ounce batch of body oil or body butter. Follow any specific instructions for the recipe you are making, as some of the recipes ask you to halve or double these blends. The Essential Oil Blends are designed, for your convenience, to be dropped directly into the recipe when called for, rather than having to pre-mix them ahead of time. If you want to mix a larger quantity to have on hand, do so in a dark-colored glass bottle with a dropper top for safe and accurate dispensing.

Most health food stores have a section of essential oils and they can easily be found online. Essential oils have varying shelf lives depending on the plant material. Generally essential oils have a shelf life of about a year, and citrus essential oils have a shorter, six-month shelf life. Patchouli and sandalwood essential oils actually improve with age. Essential oils can be stored in the refrigerator to extend the shelf life, but warm to room temperature before using them in a blend or recipe.

Essential oils are highly concentrated aromatic compounds extracted from seeds, bark, stems, roots, flowers, and other parts of plants. These phytochemicals are extracted by steam distilling or cold-pressing large amounts of plant material to extract its aromatic essence.

Less is more with essential oils, as it can take up to several pounds to create just one ounce of essential oil, so even a single drop is quite potent. As highly concentrated substances, they should be handled with care. Keep their lids on tightly or they will evaporate quickly and lose potency. Follow any usage and safety guidelines on the label. Do not use them undiluted on your skin, keep away from mucus membranes, and do not get them in your eyes. Wipe up any spills immediately and keep them away from pets and children. If you do get undiluted essential oil on your skin, apply a little olive oil to the area and wipe off. If you develop any irritation, discontinue use and consult a doctor if necessary. Pregnant women should consult their doctor about what is safe for their individual needs.

- **Sweet Citrus:** 8 drops chamomile, 24 drops lemon, 34 drops sweet orange, 20 drops lime

- **Sunny Day:** 10 drops chamomile, 32 drops sweet orange, 20 drops lemon, 18 drops lavender

- **Herby Herb:** 18 drops rosemary, 30 drops lavender, 16 drops tea tree, 18 drops peppermint

- **Pretty Flowers:** 30 drops sweet orange, 30 drops rose geranium, 20 drops ylang-ylang

- **Hippie Love:** 24 drops patchouli, 24 drops lavender, 30 drops sweet orange

- **Herbal Luxe:** 20 drops rosemary, 10 drops cardamom, 10 drops patchouli, 30 drops lemon

- **Freshness:** 28 drops peppermint, 20 drops eucalyptus, 30 drops lemon

- **Lavender Lovely:** 90 drops lavender

- **Minty:** 45 drops spearmint, 30 drops peppermint

BONUS FACIAL TREATMENTS

In this appendix you will find three detailed facial care plans, each with five steps, including facial cleanser, herbal steam, toner, mask, and moisturizer. Follow the fun and easy steps laid out for a thorough home spa facial treatment specifically for your skin type comprised of recipes from this book along with detailed instructions and helpful hints on how to use them together. Use the Bye-Bye Blackhead Treatment plan weekly to help combat congested skin. Dry and maturing skin types will love the Intensive Moisture Elixir Facial plan, which infuses healing moisture for a supple, youthful glow. The Soothing Sensitive Spa Facial will calm and replenish easily irritated skin. With these easy to follow facial care treatment guides, beautiful skin is definitely in your future!

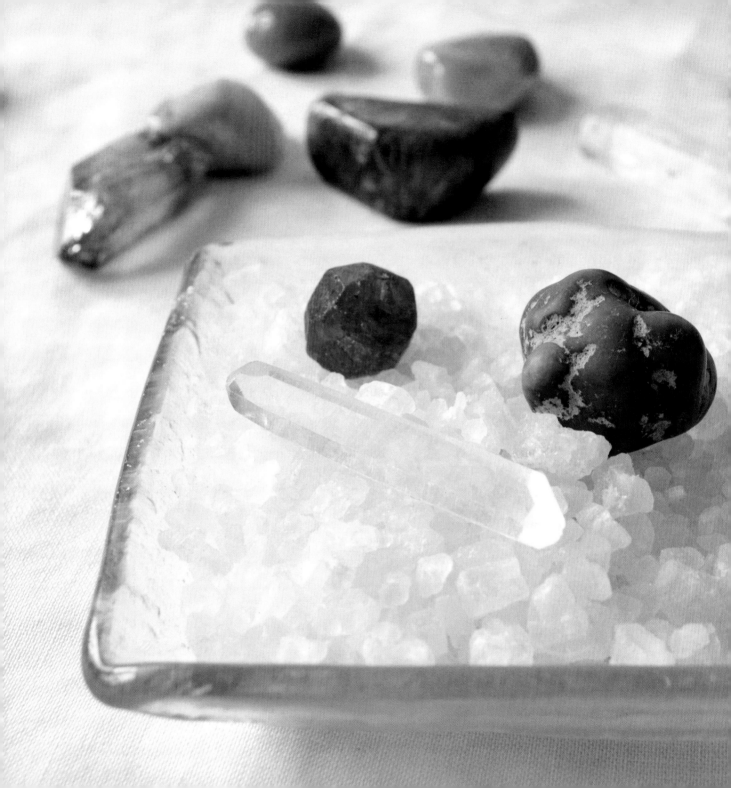

Bye-Bye Blackhead Treatment

This home spa facial was designed for skin types that are out of balance, prone to acne, blackheads, clogged pores, and irritation.

1. **Gentle Glow Washing Grains (see Chapter 2):** You get the most out of a facial when you start with a clean face. Use a mild cleanser such as the Gentle Glow Washing Grains or your usual daily cleanser. This lightly exfoliating cleanser will remove surface dirt and dead skin, enabling the steam to better penetrate and clean out any clogged pores. Use a light touch with the cleansing grains so as not to exacerbate open wounds or cystic acne.

2. **Facial Steam:** Choose the appropriate facial steam formula from Chapter 2 for your skin type and follow the directions to prepare the steam. As you're waiting for the water to boil and the herbs to steep, prepare the mask below. Remember, facial steams are designed to bring toxins to the surface. While it may initially be undesirable to "invite" this circumstance into being, it is for the best! Any underground pimples that come up were already there. A necessary step in achieving clearer skin is to bring those out, heal them quickly, and prevent any future pimples from forming.

3. **Manuka and Parsley Lightening Acne Mask (see Chapter 3):** As your pores will be quite open from the facial steam, the lemon juice in the mask may sting a bit. To avoid this, swap in the Layered Lavender Flower Water from Chapter 7, lavender hydrosol, or brewed green tea for the lemon. The substitution will only slightly reduce the lightening properties of the mask. Prepare the mask so it's ready and waiting for you when you're done with the steam. Splash your face with warm water to remove the sweat and toxins released from your pores during the steam, pat dry, and apply the mask, following the mask directions from the recipe.

4. **Facial Toner:** Using a facial toner is especially important for acne-prone skin, and even more so after performing a steam and a mask. You've just opened your pores and cleaned them out, and now it's time to close those pores to not let the gunk back in. Saturate a cotton ball with toner and gently wipe your face in an upward and outward direction. You can use the Clarifying Toner (see Chapter 2), the Layered Lavender Flower Water (see Chapter 7), or your favorite toner.

5. **Balancing Facial Moisturizer (see Chapter 2):** After an intensive facial, you want to use a mild, ultra-nourishing moisturizer that is high in antioxidants to soothe, hydrate, and protect the skin. In the four previous steps you have thoroughly cleaned and exfoliated; steamed out embedded toxins, dirt, and clogged pores; reset the pH balance; and closed your pores. This final layer of moisturizer gives a solid dose of botanical healing, like the icing on the cake. Your skin is primed to absorb high amounts of beneficial nutrients. A moisturizer calms any irritation and restores the perfect balance of moisture to your skin, creating a protective barrier to lock in the benefits from your home spa facial. Use the Balancing Facial Moisturizer or your favorite moisturizer.

Now that you've had your facial, you are beautifully content, relaxed in mind and body, smiling at your dewy, radiant, and lovely face in the mirror. You are so beautiful.

Intensive Moisture Elixir Facial

This home spa facial treatment plan is highly beneficial for skin in need of hydration and advanced nutrients, including sensitive, maturing, overexposed, sun-damaged, dry, or easily irritated skin.

❶ Gentle Glow Washing Grains (see Chapter 2): You get the most out of a facial when you start with a clean face. Use a mild cleanser such as the Gentle Glow Washing Grains or your usual daily cleanser. This lightly exfoliating cleanser will remove surface dirt and dead skin, enabling the steam to better penetrate and clean out any clogged pores.

❷ Soothing Herbal Steam (see Chapter 2): Follow the directions from the recipe to prepare the steam. As you're waiting for the water to boil and the herbs to steep, you can prepare the mask below. Boil enough water to use some to steep the yerba mate for the mask.

❸ Rainforest Elixir Mask (see Chapter 3): Directly after the facial steam, when your pores are clean and open, is the perfect time for a facial mask. Prepare the mask so it's ready and waiting for you when you're done with the steam. Splash your face with warm water to remove the sweat and toxins from the steam, pat dry, and apply the mask. The Rainforest Elixir Mask is full of superfoods and medicinal plants just packed with vital nutrients for your skin. Refrigerate the mask for an added sensory experience, and follow the mask directions from the recipe.

❹ Rooibos Rose Toner (see Chapter 2): Using a facial toner is especially important after performing a steam and a mask. You've just opened your pores and cleaned them out, and now it's time to close those pores so the gunk can't get back in. Saturate a cotton ball with toner and gently wipe your face in an upward and outward direction. You can use the Rooibos Rose Toner, Old-Fashioned Rosewater (see Chapter 7), coconut water, or your favorite toner.

❺ Vital Facial Moisturizer (see Chapter 2): After an intensive facial, you want to use a mild, ultra-nourishing moisturizer high in antioxidants to soothe, hydrate, and protect the skin. In the four previous steps you have thoroughly cleaned and exfoliated; steamed out embedded toxins, dirt, and clogged pores; reset the pH balance; and closed your pores. This final layer of moisturizer gives a solid dose of botanical healing, like the icing on the cake. Your skin is primed to absorb high amounts of beneficial nutrients. A moisturizer calms any irritation and restores the perfect balance of moisture to your skin, creating a protective barrier to lock in the benefits from your home spa facial. Use the Vital Facial Moisturizer or your favorite moisturizer.

Now that you've had your facial, you are beautifully content, relaxed in mind and body, smiling at your dewy, radiant, and lovely face in the mirror. You are so beautiful.

Soothing Sensitive Spa Facial

This is a home spa facial treatment using recipes found throughout the book. This treatment is highly beneficial for all skin types, especially sensitive, maturing, or easily irritated skin prone to redness.

1 **Gentle Glow Washing Grains (see Chapter 2):** You get the most out of a facial when you start with a clean face. Use a mild cleanser such as the Gentle Glow Washing Grains or your usual daily cleanser. This lightly exfoliating cleanser will remove surface dirt and dead skin, enabling the steam to better penetrate and clean out any clogged pores.

2 **Soothing Herbal Steam (see Chapter 2):** Follow the directions from the recipe to prepare the steam. As you're waiting for the water to boil and the herbs to steep, you can prepare the mask below.

3 **Fresh Petals Mask (see Chapter 3):** Directly after a facial steam, when your pores are clean and open, is the perfect time for a facial mask. Prepare the mask so it's ready and waiting for you when you're done with the steam. Splash your face with warm water to remove the sweat, pat dry, and apply the mask. The Fresh Petals Mask is a soothing, protein-rich, anti-inflammatory combination of fresh ingredients. Refrigerate the mask for an added sensory experience, and follow the mask directions from the recipe.

4 **Rooibos Rose Toner (see Chapter 2):** Using a facial toner is especially important after performing a steam and a mask. You've just opened your pores and cleaned them out, and now it's time to close those pores so the gunk can't get back in. Saturate a cotton ball with toner and gently wipe your face in an upward and outward direction. You can use the Rooibos Rose Toner, Old-Fashioned Rosewater (see Chapter 7), coconut water, or your favorite toner.

5 **Luxurious Vita-E Facial Oil (see Chapter 2):** After an intensive facial, you want to use a mild, ultra-nourishing moisturizer high in antioxidants to soothe, hydrate, and protect the skin. In the four previous steps you have thoroughly cleaned and exfoliated; steamed out embedded toxins, dirt, and clogged pores; reset the pH balance; and closed your pores. This final layer of moisturizer gives a solid dose of botanical healing, like the icing on the cake. Your skin is primed to absorb high amounts of beneficial nutrients. A moisturizer calms any irritation and restores the perfect balance of moisture to your skin, creating a protective barrier to lock in the benefits from your home spa facial. Use the Luxurious Vita-E Facial Oil or your favorite moisturizer.

Now that you've had your facial, you are beautifully content, relaxed in mind and body, smiling at your dewy, radiant, and lovely face in the mirror. You are so beautiful.

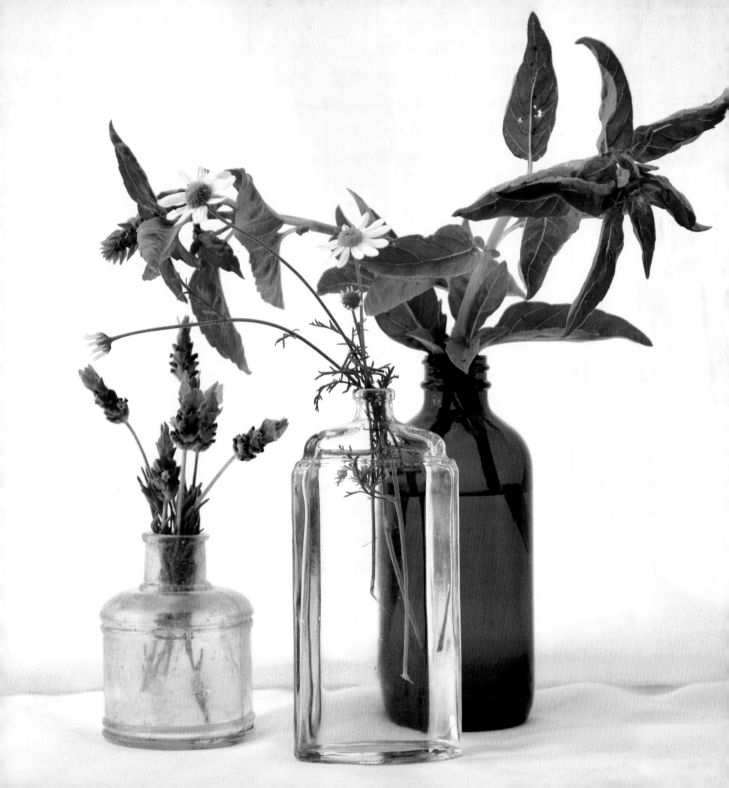

APPENDIX C

GLOSSARY OF INGREDIENTS

Acai berry: The acai berry is a reddish-purple fruit from the acai palm tree, native to Central and South America. Acai berries have a remarkable concentration of trace minerals, amino acids, essential fatty acids, phytosterols, and antioxidants. With 10 times more antioxidants than red grapes and 10–30 times the anthocyanins of red wine, acai helps combat premature aging, increases blood flow to the skin, and feeds the skin high concentrations of nutrients, which improves skin tone, texture, and radiance.

Agave: This is a natural humectant with antibacterial properties that contains trace amounts of calcium, potassium, and magnesium.

Aloe vera: Known for its healing, soothing, antibacterial, and moisturizing properties, naturally cooling aloe vera is used to relieve burning, itching, irritated skin. Recent studies indicate that aloe vera has the ability to accelerate skin cell growth.

Apple cider vinegar: This contains natural alpha-hydroxy acids, which help slough off built-up oil, grime, and dead skin cells. Apple cider vinegar contains acetic acid, which is one of the components of pain relief medications such as aspirin, making it beneficial for itchy and painful skin conditions. When topically applied, apple cider vinegar balances your skin's pH, shrinks pore size, and works to lighten discolorations, including sun and age spots.

Avocado and avocado oil: Highly moisturizing, readily absorbed, regenerative, and anti-inflammatory for the skin, avocado is high in beneficial fats, vitamins A, B_1, B_2, D, and E, minerals, and pantothenic acid. It also has high amounts of beneficial phytonutrients, including chlorophyll, omega-3 and -9 fatty acids, all of which aid in skin regeneration. It also improves the health and vitality of all skin types, including dry skin, maturing skin, sun-damaged skin, and sensitive skin.

Baking soda: Baking soda naturally cleanses your skin, washing away oil and perspiration. Baking soda is known to calm itchy skin conditions, and when added to a bath, it softens the bath water, leaving your skin silky soft.

Basil: With antibacterial properties, basil is beneficial for acne-prone skin. It can help relieve stress, headaches, and symptoms of PMS.

Beeswax: With a mild, sweet, honey-like aroma, beeswax is a natural secretion of honeybees. Beeswax is used in skin care products to thicken lip balms, butters, and salves. Beeswax adds protective, emollient, humectant, and softening elements to skin care formulations.

Black tea, *see* **Tea (black, green, and white)**

Blueberries: High in natural antioxidants, blueberries are a tannin-rich superfruit high in omega-3 fatty acids, tocopherols, carotenoids, and alpha linolenic acid. Topically applied, the fresh fruit is nourishing, calming, and astringent, while the potent antioxidants and phytonutrients are absorbed into your cells to scavenge free radicals to help slow the aging process.

Brown rice flour: Brown rice flour contains beneficial proteins, vitamins, minerals, and more than 70 antioxidants known for skin healing properties and anti-aging benefits. Brown rice cleanses pores of dirt and debris while it smoothes and softens the skin. Beneficial for all skin types, including maturing and acne prone.

Cardamom: Beneficial for muscle spasms, sinus headaches, and fatigue, cardamom's properties are warming, uplifting, refreshing, and invigorating. Cardamom's scent is fresh, sweet, green, spicy, and citrusy.

Carrot: Carrots can tone and clarify your skin, since they are naturally antiseptic and packed with antioxidants, vitamins A, B_6, C, E, and K plus folate, manganese, pantothenic acid, potassium, iron, and copper. Topically applied, carrots can be healing and rejuvenating for your skin cells.

Carrot seed essential oil: This oil revitalizes and tones the skin and is considered to be one of the best essential oils for mature skin. Carrot seed oil assists in removing toxins and water buildup in the skin, giving it a fresher, firmer appearance. It is helpful for arthritis, gout, edema, rheumatism, and conditions that cause the accumulation of toxins in muscles and joints. Carrot seed oil is known to stimulate cell growth and encourage the repair of damaged skin. Carrots are balancing for both dry and oily skin.

Castor oil: Castor oil is a very thick, rich, detoxifying, and sudsy carrier oil that attracts the dirt and toxins from your pores like a magnet, helping to carry them away. Castor oil creates a soothing, protective barrier on the skin.

Chamomile: Chamomile is a wonder herb that is universally soothing, healing, calming, relaxing, regenerative, and anti-inflammatory. A sedative to the central nervous system, chamomile helps relieve cramps, muscle spasms, PMS, menopause, headaches, hyperactivity, eczema, skin rashes, acne, cystic acne, rosacea, allergic reactions, varicose veins, and cellulite. Chamomile relaxes the mind and body when stressed, anxious, nervous, depressed, or suffering from insomnia. It brightens and brings out highlights of hair. Its analgesic action eases arthritis, lower back pain and muscle pain, rheumatism, sprains, and inflamed joints. This beautiful, magical herb gives patience and peace to mind, body, and spirit. Chamomile is great for all skin conditions, including hypersensitive skin.

Chia seeds: These are a nutrient-dense, protein-rich superfood that contains calcium, phosphorus, magnesium, manganese, copper, iron, molybdenum, niacin, zinc, and the trace mineral boron. Chia seeds are comprised of over 60 percent essential fatty acids and are the best known plant source for omega-3 fatty acids. Topically applied, chia seeds moisturize, calming the skin to soothe redness.

Chickpea flour: A common ingredient used in traditional Indian skin care as an exfoliant. Chickpea flour is known to be rejuvenating for dull, lifeless skin, to soak up oil on the skin's surface, to help unclog pores, and to clear up acne.

Cinnamon: Rich in antioxidants, cinnamon is a wonderful skin care ingredient with both anti-aging and anti-acne benefits. Research indicates that cinnamon improves collagen production in skin cells. Increased collagen helps reduce visible signs of aging. Antibacterial and anti-inflammatory, cinnamon fights acne by drying out the affected area and bringing blood and oxygen to the surface to open and unclog pores.

Cocoa butter: Cocoa butter is the solid fat expressed from the roasted seed of the cocoa seed. Cocoa butter is a soothing, antioxidant-rich emollient that has been used in skin care for centuries to heal and moisturize skin that has been exposed to the elements. High in vitamin E, it helps reduce the formation of stretch marks and scars by keeping the skin soft and supple. Cocoa butter has a shelf life of 2 to 5 years.

Cocoa powder: Cocoa is richer in antioxidants than red wine or green tea, and it gives your skin an extra boost of protection against free radicals. It is beneficial for all skin types, especially overexposed, sun-damaged, and maturing skin. Cocoa powder has rich mineral content, including calcium, potassium, and zinc along with skin-firming caffeine and theobromine.

Coconut cream: Coconut cream is full-fat coconut milk. See Coconut milk.

Coconut flour: Dried, defatted coconut makes a high-fiber, protein-rich flour when ground.

Coconut milk: Coconut milk contains vitamins C, E, B_1, B_3, B_5, and B_6 as well as iron, selenium, copper, sodium, calcium, magnesium, and phosphorus. The rich fat content in coconut milk locks moisture into the skin, and its high selenium content works to control free radicals, which helps slow down the aging process.

Coconut oil: This oil is readily absorbed into the skin and is widely known for its superior moisturizing and restorative abilities. Coconut oil is naturally full of antioxidants, has natural antifungal properties, and is an excellent moisturizer for dry, irritated, or sensitive skin.

Coconut water: Coconut water helps with increased circulation and is hydrating, high in antioxidants, and a rich source of manganese, which acts as an anti-inflammatory and helps the skin to absorb vitamins and nutrients. Fresh coconut water contains naturally occurring electrolytes.

Comfrey: Comfrey is high in allantoin, which encourages the rapid regeneration of skin cells and connective tissues and helps relieve all manner of inflammation. Additionally, comfrey contains many beneficial vitamins and nutrients, including vitamin B_{12}, protein, zinc, tannins, rosmarinic acid, and carotenes.

Cornmeal: Corn is high in the antioxidant vitamins A and C, which help the skin regenerate and fight off free radicals. It contains phytic acid, a phytochemicals that lightens and brightens skin tone. The cornmeal acts as a sponge, absorbing the oil from skin without drying it out—leaving skin soft and shine-free with radiant vitality.

Cucumber: Cucumbers are naturally cooling and have an extraordinarily soothing effect on the skin. Cucumbers are one of nature's best-known anti-inflammatory botanicals for topical use. Cucumbers contain amino acids and minerals, which help to firm and regenerate your cells.

Epsom salts: Epsom salts support stress reduction and soothe sore muscles. Epsom salts are a natural emollient that is rich in the essential mineral magnesium, which is the second most abundant element in our cells and the fourth most important positively charged ion in the body. Bathing in and exfoliating with Epsom salts are known to draw toxins from the body, sedate the nervous system, reduce pain and swelling, and relax sore muscles.

Eucalyptus essential oil: The fresh, healing aroma of eucalyptus is clean, crisp, camphoraceous, and herbaceous with soft wood undertones. Aromatherapists use eucalyptus to relieve headaches, mental exhaustion, and muscular aches and pains and to ease respiratory ailments, including colds and congestion.

Extra virgin olive oil (EVOO): EVOO is easily absorbed by the skin and is high in polyphenols, which have major anti-aging benefits. EVOO is very gentle, has many antioxidant properties, and is moisturizing, soothing, and healing to all skin types. Topically applied, EVOO helps reduce the signs of aging by absorbing UV radiation, assisting in cellular repair, and working to prevent cell damage.

Flaxseeds and flaxseed oil: Highly emollient, rich in essential fatty acids, nourishing, and skin-regenerative, flaxseeds and flaxseed oil contain vitamins A, E, and F. Flax is known to soften fine lines and aid in skin conditions such as acne, psoriasis, rosacea, and eczema. The ground seeds also possess exfoliating properties.

Ginger: Ginger is warming, soothing, and relaxing to mind, body, and spirit. It is a natural antioxidant that fights inflammation, improves circulation, and invigorates the skin to reduce the appearance and formation of cellulite, promoting a smoother, more radiant skin tone.

Grapeseed oil: Easily absorbed, this lightweight, noncomedogenic, mildly astringent, anti-inflammatory, and antiseptic oil has a silky smooth texture. It is extremely high in the antioxidant vitamins C and E and rich in oleic, linoleic, palmitic, and stearic fatty acids, which help the skin maintain moisture balance by protecting it from moisture loss. Grapeseed oil contains the amazingly strong antioxidant flavonoid oligomeric procyanidin, which is close to 50 times more powerful than vitamins A and E.

Green clay: A very fine, highly absorbent clay that soaks out oils, toxic substances, and impurities from your skin. Its toning action stimulates the skin by bringing fresh blood to damaged skin cells, revitalizing the complexion, and tightening pores. Green clay contains a plethora of trace minerals such as silica, aluminum, magnesium, calcium, iron, phosphorus, sodium, potassium, copper, zinc, selenium, cobalt, manganese, phosphorous, and silicon as well as micro-algaes, kelp, and phytonutrients.

Green tea, *see* **Tea (black, green, and white)**

Hazelnut oil: Highly beneficial for oily and acne-prone skin, hazelnut oil is light-weight with deeply penetrating astringent properties that help to tone and tighten all skin types. Hazelnut oil leaves a nongreasy feeling perfect for massage and aromatherapy. It is high in the essential fatty acids and is soothing and healing to dry, irritated skin.

Hibiscus: Hibiscus is very high in vitamin C, emollient, and astringent, which make it a beneficial ingredient in anti-aging products. It has been used in India and Asia for centuries in hair and skin care for its smoothing, calming, and firming properties.

Honey: Honey increases circulation, encouraging a natural, healthy radiance. A natural humectant, honey helps your skin absorb and retain moisture, which keeps it from drying out while keeping it glowing radiantly. Honey is packed with natural antioxidants and antimicrobial properties, which help protect, repair, and prevent skin damage.

Jojoba oil: Jojoba is not actually oil, but rather, a noncomedogenic liquid wax. It is widely considered to be one of the best choices for facial care, as it closely resembles our sebum, is highly penetrating, and does not leave an oily residue, which makes it beneficial in all types of skin care. Jojoba contains the anti-inflammatory myristic acid, which makes it a good choice to use in products formulated to relieve sore muscles, joints, and arthritis.

Kaolin clay: A white powdered form of hydrated aluminum silicate, kaolin clay has electromagnetic qualities and contains various trace minerals, including iron, magnesium, calcium, sodium, zinc, and more. The molecules in natural clays have a negative ionic surface charge that actually pulls toxins out through the pores of the skin. Kaolin is highly absorbent, drawing excess oils, impurities, and environmental toxins from the skin's surface. Clay masks dislodge old sebum that is clogged in pores.

Lavender: This universally healing herb is beneficial in skin care, as it works to regulate sebum production, fosters the regeneration of new skin cells, and soothes inflamed skin. Known to be cooling, healing, and tonic, lavender is both relaxing and revitalizing for your mind, body, and spirit. It is an adaptogen, which means that it works with your body's specific needs, adapting itself to be soothing or revitalizing as needed.

Lemon: Lemon juice adds astringent properties to fresh skin care products and helps balance oil production, reduce pimples, lighten skin, and promote healing for acne scars. Lemon essential oil works to strengthen the epidermis and stimulates the formation of connective tissue, elastin, and collagen.

Lime: A super-antioxidant fruit that increases circulation by encouraging detoxification, lime is naturally antibacterial and helps treat eczema and cellulite. Lime acts as an astringent on skin and is known to help clear oily skin. The uplifting, cheerful, and revitalizing scent of lime is known to be beneficial for sufferers of insomnia, depression, and anxiety.

Maca: Maca is a South American superfood containing iron, manganese, copper, selenium, magnesium, calcium, potassium, and iodine, plus a number of beneficial sterols. Maca is high in essential fatty acids, including linolenic acid, palmitic acid, and oleic acids as well as 19 amino acids. Topically applied, maca helps keep skin healthy by strengthening the connective tissues and fortifying the layers of the skin. Maca increases the skin's vitality, helping maintain a more youthful, wrinkle-free appearance.

Milk: Milk helps reduce redness, soothes irritated skin, and is hydrating for all skin types. Milk contains the proteins whey and casein in addition to fat, amino acids, lactic acid, and vitamins A, D, and E. These naturally occurring nutrients calm dry, itchy, upset skin and are also exfoliating and cleansing. Milk baths can help soothe dry conditions such as eczema and psoriasis.

Oat flour and oatmeal: Used for centuries as a skin soother, oatmeal nourishes, moisturizes, and gently exfoliates all skin types. Oats contain avenanthramides, flavonoids, and phenols, which are natural anti-inflammatories and antioxidants. Oatmeal can help normalize your skin's pH, which makes it especially helpful for soothing irritated skin conditions. Oats make an effective natural cleanser due to saponins, which absorb dirt, oil, and odor.

Orange zest and juice: High in vitamin C, potassium, folic acid, and naturally occurring alpha-hydroxy acids, oranges are clinically proven to prevent wrinkles and fine lines. Topically applied, orange is known to reduce blemishes, help fade dark spots, and improve the overall texture and color of the skin. Orange is an exfoliant and works against the premature aging of skin by stimulating new cell production, promoting increased collagen levels, and encouraging firm skin. It's good for blemished, oily, and acne-prone skin.

Oregano: Oregano is an aromatic herb with high levels of antioxidants that boasts antifungal, antiviral, anti-aging, antibacterial, anti-inflammatory, and antiparasitic properties. It helps relieve the symptoms of arthritis, rheumatism, and sore muscles as well as aiding skin conditions such as psoriasis and eczema.

Parsley: With more vitamin C than citrus fruits, parsley is well known for its skin-lightening properties that help reduce the appearance of dark spots and discoloration. When topically applied, parsley is known to help reduce inflammation, curb acne outbreaks, and heal existing blemishes.

Patchouli essential oil: Patchouli essential oil is a skin conditioner with antiseptic, antifungal, antibacterial properties, which make it helpful for healing dry skin, eczema, acne, and inflamed or cracked skin conditions. Patchouli is known to rejuvenate skin cells, help reduce enlarged pores, and help relieve skin discolorations. Additionally, aromatherapists use it for headache relief, for stress-related disorders, and as an antidepressant.

Peppermint leaves and essential oil: Peppermint is known to be both soothing and stimulating, and its anti-inflammatory properties help calm irritated skin. Peppermint oil may also contain some sun protection properties.

Pineapple: Pineapple is a tropical fruit that is a natural antioxidant high in vitamin C. It is an exfoliant due to a protein-digesting enzyme called bromelain, and it has proteolytic enzymes, which help stimulate and cleanse inflamed, sore skin. Applied topically, pineapple is known to stimulate collagen production, fight free radicals, and help reduce the appearance of age spots and fine lines.

Pink grapefruit essential oil: This essential oil's uplifting scent is said to help relieve depression, mental exhaustion, and headaches. Pink grapefruit essential oil helps fight against cellulite, muscle fatigue, fluid retention, and toxins. In skin care, it is used for congested, oily, and acne-prone skin due to its tonic, astringent, and antibacterial properties.

Poppy seeds: High in linoleic acid and omega-3 fatty acids, poppy seeds are an effective natural exfoliator.

Pumpkin: Pumpkin is rich in alpha-hydroxy acids, which makes it a great enzymatic exfoliator. Anti-inflammatory pumpkin contains more than 100 "skin food" nutrients and essential fatty acids—including beta carotene, vitamin A, and zinc—that are known to stimulate circulation, increase cellular renewal, and promote healing, helping reverse the signs of aging. The high levels of natural antioxidants in pumpkin work to effectively protect against free radical damage, and its high levels of the antioxidant vitamin C work to brighten the skin and even out pigmentation. Pumpkin also helps to regulate oil production and reduce the size and appearance of your pores.

Red raspberry seed oil: An excellent oil to enhance protection against the sun, red raspberry seed oil has a high content of essential fatty acids and tocopherols, which nourish and hydrate the skin, leaving it soft and smooth. Studies have shown that Red Raspberry Seed Oil contains sun protection properties ranging from SPF 28–50.

Red wine: Red wine has 20 to 50 times the antioxidant power of vitamins E and C, and it contains powerful anti-aging nutrients like resveratrol, which has anticancer effects. Topical application of red wine helps fight off free radical attacks and is perfect for all skin types, especially for maturing, sun-damaged, and overexposed skin.

Rooibos: Rooibos is a powerful antioxidant that has high levels of vitamins and minerals, including vitamin D and zinc. Japanese scientists have discovered that rooibos tea contains a mimic of the enzyme superoxide dismutase (SOD), an amazing antioxidant that attacks free radicals, thereby limiting their damaging effects on our skin. Beneficial for all skin types, rooibos is hypoallergenic and antibacterial.

Rose: Known to be highly emollient, rose helps fight premature aging and improves tone, texture, and elasticity. Anti-inflammatory and antibacterial, rose is soothing, balancing, and refreshing, making it beneficial for all skin types and conditions. Aromatherapists believe the scent of rose to be calming and soothing to the mind and spirit. Rose is also an aphrodisiac and a balm to the heart.

Rose geranium essential oil: Rose geranium essential oil helps to tone skin tissues, aids in cell regeneration and tissue repair, and works to reduce cellulite, dermatitis, and eczema. Astringent, antiseptic, antifungal, anti-infectious, antibacterial, anti-inflammatory, and regenerative, this essential oil is known to help with aged or wrinkling skin, cellular regeneration, and acne. It's also antiseptic and good for both dry and oily skin.

Rosemary: A robust, detoxifying herb, rosemary helps relieve a wide variety of ailments, including hangovers, irritability, tension, headaches, liver problems, muscular pain, rheumatism, poor circulation, cellulite, stress, and more. Beneficial in skin care preparations for its wrinkle-smoothing, antibacterial, and oil-regulating properties, rosemary is historically known to stimulate the conscious mind, improving concentration, mental clarity, and memory. It is beneficial in stimulating hair growth and helps relieve dry, itchy scalp conditions such as dandruff.

Rosewater: Used in skin care preparations for centuries, rosewater is naturally astringent and antiseptic. It helps tighten pores, soothe capillaries, reduce redness, fight blemishes, smooth wrinkles, and restore suppleness for a dewy complexion. Rosewater soothes irritated skin conditions, including acne, sunburn, or overexposure to the elements and is beneficial for all skin types, including dry, oily, and sensitive.

Sea salt: Solar-dried sea salts retain the rich vitamins, minerals, trace elements, and amino acids of the sea. Sea salts have a very high concentration of calcium, magnesium, potassium, sodium, and bromide that are essential for healthy-looking skin and naturally alleviate redness, irritation, and swelling due to blemished skin. Sea salt baths and body scrubs are believed to increase circulation and bring more white blood cells toward the surface of your skin, helping to heal imperfections and giving your skin a natural glow. In effect, the skin is tightened and the appearance of pores, cellulite, wrinkles, and lines can be reduced.

Shea butter: With an abundance of healing properties and superior moisturizing capability, shea butter actually restores the skin's natural elasticity. Shea butter contains a ton of naturally occurring healing elements, including vitamins, minerals, proteins, and a unique fatty acid profile. Shea butter enables your skin to absorb moisture from the air, and as a result, your skin becomes softer and stays moisturized for longer. Shea butter has a natural sun protection ranging between SPF 6–7.

Soy milk: Rich in isoflavones and vitamins, soy milk is beneficial in skin care to reduce the appearance of fine lines and wrinkles.

Spirulina: Spirulina is an iron-rich blue-green algae superfood that is 65 percent amino acids and high in essential fatty acids, vitamins, and nutrients, including beta carotene, chlorophyll, and calcium. Spirulina contains significant amounts of the powerhouse antioxidant superoxide dismutase (SOD) that attacks free radicals, thereby limiting their damaging effects on your skin.

Strawberries: This superfruit is high in polyphenols and highly anti-inflammatory due to an amazing combination of beneficial phytonutrients, including anthocyanins, ellagitannins, flavonols, terpenoids, phenolic acid, and vitamin C. Due to their salicylic acid and alpha-hydroxy acid content, strawberries are brightening and exfoliating and promote clear skin and a youthful glow.

Sugar: Sugar is a great natural exfoliator due to its texture and glycolic acid content, which allows for effective yet gentle abrasion. Glycolic acids help cleanse pores and improve overall skin tone and texture by removing dead, dull skin cells.

Sweet almond oil: Rich in beneficial vitamins and minerals—including vitamins A, B_1, B_3, B_6, E, and D, plus magnesium and calcium—sweet almond oil is a lightweight, satiny-smooth, easily absorbed oil that has little or no scent. Sweet almond oil is anti-inflammatory and beneficial for all skin types and helps to relieve dry skin and irritated skin.

Sweet orange essential oil: This sweet, fruity, joyful, and uplifting oil is considered a stress reliever and an antidepressant. Sweet orange essential oil is anti-inflammatory, antiseptic, and detoxifying. In skin care it strengthens the epidermis, increases collagen production, improves circulation, and soothes dry and irritated skin.

Tea (black, green, and white): Black, green, and white teas all come from the Camellia sinensis plant but are picked at different times. White tea leaves are picked early on as young leaf sprouts, green tea is picked midmaturation, and black tea comes from the mature leaves and is often aged or roasted to deepen the flavor and aroma. Tea is a powerful antioxidant and may be used topically or internally as a tea before or after sun exposure. Tea has been shown to help reduce skin inflammation, calm redness, protect skin cells, and assist with the adverse effects of UV radiation exposure. It naturally contains tannic acid, theobromine, and polyphenols—all of which are soothing and healing to sunburned and environmentally damaged skin.

Tea tree essential oil: Tea tree oil is prized for its powerful antibacterial, antifungal, antiseptic, and antiviral properties. It destroys bacteria and helps heal acne, psoriasis, eczema, and many other conditions, including bug bites, cuts, and burns. Tea tree essential oil also benefits the immune and endocrine systems.

Thyme: This antioxidant herb boosts circulation and has antibacterial properties. It is beneficial for acne-prone skin and helps fade acne scars as well as age spots.

Turbinado sugar: This is a coarse-grained, and unrefined, dark brown sugar that is less processed—and healthier—than regular sugar. Being less processed means that turbinado sugar retains more nutrients of the cane juice as well as naturally occurring glycolic acids (see Sugar for more information).

Turmeric: Anti-inflammatory, antioxidant, antiseptic, and astringent, turmeric provides texture in exfoliation recipes and helps fight wrinkles for a more youthful appearance. Beneficial for acneic skin, turmeric works to regulate oil production and helps fade acne scars. Undiluted turmeric will stain the skin.

Vitamin E: This vitamin protects skin cells and membranes from environmental damage caused by UV rays, pollutants, and aging. Although vitamin E is a thick concentrated oily substance, it allows the skin to breathe and function naturally. Vitamin E helps to reduce the appearance of wrinkles and the formation of scar tissue, and it can also be used as an antioxidant to help sustain shelf life of products containing botanical oils.

White tea, *see* **Tea (black, green, and white)**

Witch hazel: A gentle, natural anti-inflammatory, antimicrobial astringent that helps tighten pores with a cool soothing sensation, witch hazel provides protection from scavenging free radicals, soothes inflamed skin, and has moisturizing properties that make it highly beneficial for all skin types and conditions. Witch hazel also protects against sun damage.

Yerba mate: Yerba mate contains 196 active chemicals, including 24 vitamins and minerals, 15 amino acids, and 11 polyphenols—a group of phytochemicals that act as powerful antioxidants. These are: vitamins A, C, E, B_1, B_2, niacin (B_3), B_5, B complex; the minerals calcium, manganese, iron, selenium, potassium, magnesium, and phosphorus; and various additional compounds, including fatty acids, chlorophyll, flavonols, polyphenols, trace minerals, antioxidants, pantothenic acid, and 15 amino acids.

Yogurt: Yogurt promotes a healthy glow for all skin types. It moisturizes and exfoliates dry skin and unclogs and reduces size of pores in oily skin. Yogurt is high in calcium, protein, vitamin D, and living probiotic organisms and is a mild exfoliant due to lactic acid, which is a natural alpha-hydroxy acid. Topically applied to the skin, yogurt is soothing, calming, and moisturizing; it helps prevent premature aging, fights acne, and works to reduce redness and discoloration.

Zinc oxide: A naturally occurring mineral that provides broad-spectrum sunscreen protection from both UVA and UVB radiation when added to a lotion or cream, zinc oxide is also often used for its soothing effects (as in diaper rash ointments) and may contain antifungal properties. Zinc physically blocks the sun's rays by reflecting UV radiation.

METRIC
CONVERSION
CHART

VOLUME CONVERSIONS

U.S. Volume Measure	Metric Equivalent
⅛ teaspoon	0.5 milliliter
¼ teaspoon	1 milliliter
½ teaspoon	2 milliliters
1 teaspoon	5 milliliters
½ tablespoon	7 milliliters
1 tablespoon (3 teaspoons)	15 milliliters
2 tablespoons (1 fluid ounce)	30 milliliters
¼ cup (4 tablespoons)	60 milliliters
⅓ cup	90 milliliters
½ cup (4 fluid ounces)	125 milliliters
⅔ cup	160 milliliters
¾ cup (6 fluid ounces)	180 milliliters
1 cup (16 tablespoons)	250 milliliters
1 pint (2 cups)	500 milliliters
1 quart (4 cups)	1 liter (about)

WEIGHT CONVERSIONS

U.S. Weight Measure	Metric Equivalent
½ ounce	15 grams
1 ounce	30 grams
2 ounces	60 grams
3 ounces	85 grams
¼ pound (4 ounces)	115 grams
½ pound (8 ounces)	225 grams
¾ pound (12 ounces)	340 grams
1 pound (16 ounces)	454 grams

INDEX

A

Acai berry, 204
Acai Berry Facial Scrub, 16
Acne mask, 55
After-sun face and body mask, 180
Agave, 204
Agave Rose Anti-Aging Mask, 58
Almond Moisture Scrub, 76–77
Aloe vera, 204
Ambrosia Face and Body Mask, 155
Angel Face Botanicals, 12
Angel Soak for Cold and Flu, 120–21
Anti-aging mask, 58
Anti-itch paste, 183
Antioxidant skin quencher, 181
Apple cider vinegar, 204
Aromatherapy, 12
Aromatic Vanilla Infusion, 146
Avocado and avocado oil, 204
Avo-Oat After-Sun Face and Body
    Mask, 180
Ayurvedic Facial Cleansing Grains, 19
Ayurvedic medicine, 12
Aztec Honey and Wine Mask, 49

B

Baking pan sizes, 215
Baking soda, 204
Balancing Facial Moisturizer, 28
Balms
    Gardener's Herbal Balm, 95
    Shea Butter Lip Balm, 17
Basil, 204
Bath Fizzies, 117–19
Bath Melts, 114–15
Bath recipes
    about: overview of, 109
    Angel Soak for Cold and Flu, 120–21
    Bath Fizzies, 117–19

Bath Melts, 114–15
Chamomile and Oat Super Soothe-
    Me Bath, 125–26
Coconut, Lime, and Rose Petals
    Bath, 110
Ideal Luxury Bath, 123–24
Mermaid Bath, 111
Moisturizing Bath Salts, 116
Soothe-My-Sunburn, 184–85
Sunshine C Bath, 112
Bath sachets, 126
Bath salts, 116
Beachy Babe Hair Spray, 192
Beeswax, 204
Blueberries, 204
Blushing Bride Ubtan Exfoliant, 157–59
Body Butter Bars, 90–91
Body butters and oils
    about: overview of recipes, 89
    Body Butter Bars, 90–91
    Coco-Spice Body Butter, 100
    Cuticle Saver Treatment, 107
    Gardener's Herbal Balm, 95
    Healing Comfrey Salve, 92
    Lovely Body Butter, 97
    Luxurious Body Oil, 102
    Sore Muscle Massage Oil, 103
    Warm Cinnamon Massage Oil, 104
    Whipped Shea Body Butter, 96
Body scrubs and washes
    about: overview of recipes, 63
    Almond Moisture Scrub, 76–77
    Citrus Blast Body Scrub, 72
    Floral Oatmeal Wash, 80–81
    Gentle Oatmeal Wash, 70
    Herb Garden Body Scrub, 69
    Honey Coconut Body Wash, 87
    Invigorating Ginger Citrus Body
        Wash, 84
    Javanese Gold Body Scrub, 65
    Lemon Poppy Seed Scrub, 83

Mocha Latte Scrub, 71
Olive Butter Scrub, 64
Shea Butter Body Wash, 86
Sugar Chai Honey Scrub, 66
Valencia Coffee Scrub, 79
Vanilla, Bourbon, and Honey Scrub,
    75
Brown rice flower, 205
Butters
    Body Butter Bars, 90
    Coco-Spice Body Butter, 100
    Lovely Body Butter, 97
Bye-Bye Blackhead Treatment, 199

C

Calming Antioxidant Skin Quencher,
    181
Cardamom, 205
Carrot, 205
Carrot seed essential oil, 205
Carrot-Coconut NutraMoist Mask, 47
Castor oil, 205
Chamomile, 205
Chamomile and Oat Super Soothe-Me
    Bath, 125–26
Chia Coconut Superfood Mask, 52
Chia seeds, 205
Chickpea flour, 205
Chocolate Lip Scrub, 37
Cinnamon, 206
Citrus Blast Body Scrub, 72
Clarifying Probiotic Moisture Surge, 46
Clarifying Toner, 22
Cleansing grains
    Ayurvedic Facial Cleansing Grains,
        19
    Green Tea and Adzuki Cleansing
        Grains, 38
Clogged pores, cleanser for, 23–25
Cocoa butter and powder, 206

Coconut, Lime, and Rose Petals Bath, 110
Coconut cantaloupe cooler, 172
Coconut cream and milk and water, 206
Coconut flower, 206
Coconut oil, 206
Coconut Rice Conditioning Exfoliant, 154
Coco-Spice Body Butter, 100
Coco-Superfruit Mask, 50
Cold and flu soak, 120–21
Comfrey, 206
Comfrey oil, 137
Comfrey salve, 92
Complements, 13
Cooling Anti-Itch Paste, 183
Cornmeal, 206
Cucumber, 207
Cucumber De-Puffer Spa Water, 169
Cucumber Rose Sunburn Relief, 189
Cuticle Saver Treatment, 107

D

Dehydration and bathing, 115
De-puffer spa water, 169
Detoxifying Seaweed Body Wrap, 160–61
Dreamtime-infused oil, 142

E

Epsom salts, 207
Essential oils
    about: overview of, 195
    in bath, 119
    blends, 195–96
Eucalyptus essential oil, 207
Exfoliants

Blushing Bride Ubtan Exfoliant, 157–59
Coconut Rice Conditioning Exfoliant, 154
Extra virgin olive oil (EVOO), 207
Eye cream, 32

F

Facial care
    about: overview of recipes, 15
    Acai Berry Facial Scrub, 16
    Ayurvedic Facial Cleansing Grains, 19
    Balancing Facial Moisturizer, 28
    Chocolate Lip Scrub, 37
    Clarifying Toner, 22
    Gentle Glow Washing Grains, 20
    Green Tea and Adzuki Cleansing Grains, 38–39
    Green Tea Eye Cream, 32
    Luxurious Vita-E Facial Oil, 31
    Maca Vitality Scrub, 18
    Oil Cleanser for Clogged Pores, 23–25
    Rooibos Rose Toner, 26
    Shea Butter Lip Balm, 17
    Soothing Herbal Steam, 34
    Spa Facial Steam for Normal to Oily Skin, 33
    steps, 15
    Vital Facial Moisturizer, 29
Facial care plans
    about: overview of treatments, 197
    Bye-Bye Blackhead Treatment, 199
    Intensive Moisture Elixir Facial, 200
    Soothing Sensitive Spa Facial, 201
Facial cleansing grains, 19

Facial masks
    about: overview of recipes, 41
    Agave Rose Anti-Aging Mask, 58
    Aztec Honey and Wine Mask, 49
    Carrot-Coconut NutraMoist Mask, 47
    Chia Coconut Superfood Mask, 52
    Clarifying Probiotic Moisture Surge, 46
    Coco-Superfruit Mask, 50
    Fresh Petals Mask, 61
    Go Green Moisture Mask, 56
    Green Clay Rose Milk Mask, 44
    Manuka and Parsley Lightening Acne Mask, 55
    Radiant Orange Mask, 43
    Rainforest Elixir Mask, 59
    Soothing Oil-Free Mask, 53
    Yerba Flax Face-Food Mask, 42
Facial moisturizers
    Balancing Facial Moisturizer, 28
    Vital Facial Moisturizer, 29
Facial steams
    Soothing Herbal Steam, 34
    Spa Facial Steam for Normal to Oily Skin, 33
Fizzies, bath, 117–19
Fizzy Mojito Foot Spa, 162
Flaxseeds and flaxseed oil, 207
Floral Oatmeal Wash, 80–81
Flower waters, 145
Foot spa, 162
Fresh Comfrey Oil, 137
Fresh Herbal Oil, 139
Fresh Petals Mask, 61
Freshness essential oil, 196

G

Gardener's Herbal Balm, 95
Gentle Glow Washing Grains, 20
Gentle Oatmeal Wash, 70
Ginger, 207
Glowing Goddess Face and Body Mask, 152
Go Green Moisture Mask, 56
Grapeseed oil, 207
Green clay, 207
Green Clay Rose Milk Mask, 44
Green moisture mask, 56
Green Tea and Adzuki Cleansing Grains, 38–39
Green Tea Eye Cream, 32
Green Tea-Infused Oil, 130–31

H

Hair finishing oil, 166
Hair spray, 192
Hazelnut oil, 208
Head-to-Toe Pumpkin Mask, 150–51
Healing Comfrey Salve, 92
Healing Sunburn Spray and Compress, 186
Healthy skin, 11, 167
Herb Garden Body Scrub, 69
Herbal balm, 95
Herbal Luxe essential oil, 196
Herbal oil, 139
Herby Herb essential oil, 196
Hibiscus, 208
Hippie Love essential oil, 196
Home spa
    about: overview of, 12–13
    "me time," 12, 13
    planning, 9
Honey, 208

Honey and wine mask, 49
Honey Coconut Body Wash, 87
Hydration
    bathing, 161
    detoxification and, 161
    healthy skin and, 167

I

Ideal Luxury Bath, 123–24
Infusions
    about: overview of recipes, 129
    Aromatic Vanilla Infusion, 146
    Fresh Comfrey Oil, 137
    Fresh Herbal Oil, 139
    Green Tea-Infused Oil, 130–31
    Lavender-Infused Oil, 140
    Layered Lavender Flower Water, 143
    Old-Fashioned Rosewater, 145
    Rosemary-Infused Oil, 133–34
    Sweet Dreamtime-Infused Oil, 142
    Thai Spice-Infused Oil, 132
    use safety, 129
    Vanilla-Infused Oil, 136
Ingredients, 9, 11–12, 203–13
Intensive Moisture Elixir Facial, 200
Invigorating Ginger Citrus Body Wash, 84

J

Jasmine Hair Finishing Oil, 166
Javanese Gold Body Scrub, 65
Jojoba oil, 208

K

Kaolin clay, 208

L

Lavender, 208
Lavender flower water, 143
Lavender Lovely essential oil, 196
Lavender-Infused Oil, 140
Layered Lavender Flower Water, 143
Lemon, 208
Lemon Poppy Seed Scrub, 83
Lime, 208
Lip balm, 17
Lip scrub, 37
Love yourself, 13
Lovely Body Butter, 97
Luxurious Body Oil, 102
Luxurious Vita-E Facial Oil, 31
Luxury bath, 123–24

M

Maca, 209
Maca Vitality Scrub, 18
Manuka and Parsley Lightening Acne Mask, 55
Masks
    Agave Rose Anti-Aging Mask, 58
    Ambrosia Face and Body Mask, 155
    Avo-Oat After-Sun Face and Body Mask, 180
    Aztec Honey and Wine Mask, 49
    Carrot-Coconut NutraMoist Mask, 47
    Chia Coconut Superfood Mask, 52
    Coco-Superfruit Mask, 50
    Fresh Petals Mask, 61
    Glowing Goddess Face and Body Mask, 152
    Go Green Moisture Mask, 56
    Green Clay Rose Milk Mask, 44
    Head-to-Toe Pumpkin Mask, 150–51

Manuka and Parsley Lightening Acne Mask, 55

Radiant Orange Mask, 43

Rainforest Elixir Mask, 59

Soothing Oil-Free Mask, 53

Yerba Flax Face-Food Mask, 42

Yogurt Lavender Comfort Body Mask and Bath, 179

Massage oils, 103, 104

Melts, bath, 114–15

Mermaid Bath, 111

Metric conversion chart, 214–15

Milk, 209

Minty essential oil, 196

Mocha Latte Scrub, 71

Moisturizers

Balancing Facial Moisturizer, 28

Vital Facial Moisturizer, 29

Moisturizing Bath Salts, 116

N

Natural skin care, 12

O

Oat flour and oatmeal, 209

Oil Cleanser for Clogged Pores, 23–25

Oil-free mask, 53

Oils

Cuticle Saver Treatment, 107

Fresh Comfrey Oil, 137

Fresh Herbal Oil, 139

Green Tea-Infused Oil, 130–31

Jasmine Hair Finishing Oil, 166

Lavender-Infused Oil, 140

Luxurious Body Oil, 102

Luxurious Vita-E Facial Oil, 31

Rosemary-Infused Oil, 133–34

Sore Muscle Massage Oil, 103

Sweet Dreamtime-Infused Oil, 142

Thai spice-infused, 132

Vanilla-Infused Oil, 136

Warm Cinnamon Massage Oil, 104

Old-Fashioned Rosewater, 145

Olive Butter Scrub, 64

Orange mask, 43

Orange zest and juice, 209

Oregano, 209

Organic skin care, 12

Oven temperature conversions, 215

P

Parsley, 209

Patchouli essential oil, 209

Peppermint leaves and essential oil, 210

Perfume, vanilla, 156

Petals mask, 61

Pineapple, 210

Pink grapefruit essential oil, 210

Poppy seeds, 210

Pre-tanning scrub, 176

Pretty Flowers essential oil, 196

Probiotic moisture surge, 46

Pumpkin, 210

Pumpkin mask, 150–51

Q

Quick Coconut Cantaloupe Cooler, 172

R

Radiant Orange Mask, 43

Rainforest Elixir Mask, 59

Rasayana, 12

Red raspberry seed oil, 9, 210

Red wine, 210

Rooibos, 210

Rooibos Rose Toner, 26

Rose, 211

Rose geranium oil, 211

Rose petals, coconut, and lime bath, 110

Rosemary, 211

Rosemary-Infused Oil, 133–34

Rosewater, 145, 211

Rosy Green Tea Spa Water, 173

S

Sachets, bath, 126

Salts, bath, 116

Salve, comfrey, 92

Scalp and hair treatment, 164–65

Scents, incorporating, 98

Scrubs, 176

Acai Berry Facial Scrub, 16

Almond Moisture Scrub, 76–77

Chocolate Lip Scrub, 37

Citrus Blast Body Scrub, 72

Herb Garden Body Scrub, 69

Javanese Gold Body Scrub, 65

Lemon Poppy Seed Scrub, 83

Maca Vitality Scrub, 18

Mocha Latte Scrub, 71

Olive Butter Scrub, 64

Sugar Chai Honey Scrub, 66

Sun-Kissed Pre-Tanning Body Scrub, 176

Valencia Coffee Scrub, 79

Vanilla, Bourbon, and Honey Scrub, 75

Sea salt, 211

Seaweed body wrap, 160–61

Shea butter, 96, 211

Shea Butter Body Wash, 86

Shea Butter Lip Balm, 17

Skin
    about: overview of, 11
    healthy, 11, 167
    hydration and, 167
Skin care. *See also* Skin care recipes
    about: overview of, 13
    herbal, 12
    natural and organic, 12
Skin care recipes
    about: baths, 109–26; body butters
        and oils, 89–107; body scrubs and
        washes, 63–87; facial care, 15–39;
        facial masks, 41–61; infusions, 129–
        46; large batch, 12; overview of, 9,
        13; single use, 12; sun care, 175–92;
        whole body spa treatments, 149–73
    Acai Berry Facial Scrub, 16
    Agave Rose Anti-Aging Mask, 58
    Almond Moisture Scrub, 76–77
    Ambrosia Face and Body Mask, 155
    Angel Soak for Cold and Flu, 120–21
    Aromatic Vanilla Infusion, 146
    Avo-Oat After-Sun Face and Body
        Mask, 180
    Ayurvedic Facial Cleansing Grains,
        19
    Aztec Honey and Wine Mask, 49
    Balancing Facial Moisturizer, 28
    Bath Fizzies, 117–19
    Bath Melts, 114–15
    Beachy Babe Hair Spray, 192
    Blushing Bride Ubtan Exfoliant,
        157–59
    Body Butter Bars, 90–91
    Calming Antioxidant Skin Quencher,
        181
    Carrot-Coconut NutraMoist Mask,
        47
    Chamomile and Oat Super Soothe-
        Me Bath, 125–26

Chia Coconut Superfood Mask, 52
Chocolate Lip Scrub, 37
Citrus Blast Body Scrub, 72
Clarifying Probiotic Moisture Surge,
    46
Clarifying Toner, 22
Coconut, Lime, and Rose Petals
    Bath, 110
Coconut Rice Conditioning
    Exfoliant, 154
Coco-Spice Body Butter, 100
Coco-Superfruit Mask, 50
Cooling Anti-Itch Paste, 183
Cucumber De-Puffer Spa Water, 169
Cucumber Rose Sunburn Relief, 189
Cuticle Saver Treatment, 107
Detoxifying Seaweed Body Wrap,
    160–61
Fizzy Mojito Foot Spa, 162
Floral Oatmeal Wash, 80–81
Fresh Comfrey Oil, 137
Fresh Herbal Oil, 139
Fresh Petals Mask, 61
Gardener's Herbal Balm, 95
Gentle Glow Washing Grains, 20
Gentle Oatmeal Wash, 70
Glowing Goddess Face and Body
    Mask, 152
Go Green Moisture Mask, 56
Green Clay Rose Milk Mask, 44
Green Tea and Adzuki Cleansing
    Grains, 38–39
Green Tea Eye Cream, 32
Green Tea-Infused Oil, 130–31
Head-to-Toe Pumpkin Mask, 150–51
Healing Comfrey Salve, 92
Healing Sunburn Spray and
    Compress, 186
Herb Garden Body Scrub, 69
Honey Coconut Body Wash, 87
Ideal Luxury Bath, 123–24

Invigorating Ginger Citrus Body
    Wash, 84
Jasmine Hair Finishing Oil, 166
Javanese Gold Body Scrub, 65
Lavender-Infused Oil, 140
Layered Lavender Flower Water, 143
Lemon Poppy Seed Scrub, 83
Lovely Body Butter, 97
Luxurious Body Oil, 102
Luxurious Vita-E Facial Oil, 31
Maca Vitality Scrub, 18
Manuka and Parsley Lightening
    Acne Mask, 55
Mermaid Bath, 111
Mocha Latte Scrub, 71
Moisturizing Bath Salts, 116
Oil Cleanser for Clogged Pores,
    23–25
Old-Fashioned Rosewater, 145
Olive Butter Scrub, 64
Quick Coconut Cantaloupe Cooler,
    172
Radiant Orange Mask, 43
Rainforest Elixir Mask, 59
Rooibos Rose Toner, 26
Rosemary-Infused Oil, 133–34
Rosy Green Tea Spa Water, 173
Shea Butter Body Wash, 86
Shea Butter Lip Balm, 19
Soothe-My-Sunburn Bath, 184–85
Soothing Herbal Steam, 34
Soothing Oil-Free Mask, 53
Soothing Scalp and Hair Treatment,
    164–65
Sore Muscle Massage Oil, 103
Spa Facial Steam for Normal to Oily
    Skin, 33
Strawberry Super C Sipper, 170
Sugar Chai Honey Scrub, 66
Sun Protection Lotion Stick, 190–91

Sun-Kissed Pre-Tanning Body
Scrub, 176
Sunrise Spa Water, 167
Sunshine C Bath, 112
Sweet Dreamtime-Infused Oil, 142
Thai Spice-Infused Oil, 132
Valencia Coffee Scrub, 79
Vanilla, Bourbon, and Honey Scrub,
75
Vanilla Isle Perfume, 156
Vanilla-Infused Oil, 136
Vital Facial Moisturizer, 29
Warm Cinnamon Massage Oil, 104
Whipped Shea Body Butter, 96
Yerba Flax Face-Food Mask, 42
Yogurt Lavender Comfort Body
Mask and Bath, 179
Soothe-me bath, 125–26
Soothe-My-Sunburn Bath, 184–85
Soothing Herbal Steam, 34
Soothing Oil-Free Mask, 53
Soothing Scalp and Hair Treatment,
164–65
Soothing Sensitive Spa Facial, 201
Sore Muscle Massage Oil, 103
Soy milk, 211
Spa Facial Steam for Normal to Oily
Skin, 33
Spa water
Cucumber De-Puffer Spa Water, 169
Rosy Green Tea Spa Water, 173
Sunrise Spa Water, 167
Spirulina, 212
Steams
Soothing Herbal Steam, 34
Spa Facial Steam for Normal to Oily
Skin, 33

Strawberries, 212
Strawberry Super C Sipper, 170
Sugar, 212
Sugar Chai Honey Scrub, 66
Sun care
about: overview of recipes, 175
Avo-Oat After-Sun Face and Body
Mask, 180
Beachy Babe Hair Spray, 192
Calming Antioxidant Skin Quencher,
181
Cooling Anti-Itch Paste, 183
Cucumber Rose Sunburn Relief, 189
Healing Sunburn Spray and
Compress, 186
Soothe-My-Sunburn Bath, 184–85
Sun Protection Lotion Stick, 190–91
Sun-Kissed Pre-Tanning Body
Scrub, 176
Yogurt Lavender Comfort Body
Mask and Bath, 179
Sun Protection Lotion Stick, 190–91
Sunburn
Cucumber Rose Sunburn Relief, 189
Healing Sunburn Spray and
Compress, 186
Soothe-My-Sunburn Bath, 184–85
Sun-Kissed Pre-Tanning Body Scrub,
176
Sunny Day essential oil, 196
Sunrise Spa Water, 167
Sunshine C Bath, 112
Super C sipper, 170
Sweet almond oil, 212
Sweet Citrus essential oil, 196
Sweet Dreamtime-Infused Oil, 142
Sweet orange essential oil, 212

T
Tea, 212
Tea tree essential oil, 212
Thai Spice-Infused Oil, 132
Thyme, 212
Toners
Clarifying Toner, 22
Rooibos Rose Toner, 26
Traditional Chinese medicine, 12
Turbinado sugar, 212
Turmeric, 213

U
Ubtan exfoliant, 157–59

V
Valencia Coffee Scrub, 79
Vanilla, Bourbon, and Honey Scrub, 75
Vanilla infusion, 146
Vanilla Isle Perfume, 156
Vanilla-Infused Oil, 136
Vita-E facial oil, 31
Vital Facial Moisturizer, 29
Vitality scrub, 18
Vitamin E, 213
Volume conversions, 215

W
Warm Cinnamon Massage Oil, 104
Washes
Floral Oatmeal Wash, 80–81
Gentle Oatmeal Wash, 70

Honey Coconut Body Wash, 87

Invigorating Ginger Citrus Body
Wash, 84

Shea Butter Body Wash, 86

Washing grains, 20

Weight conversions, 215

Whipped Shea Body Butter, 96

Whole body spa treatments

about: overview of recipes, 149

Ambrosia Face and Body Mask, 155

Blushing Bride Ubtan Exfoliant,
157–59

Coconut Rice Conditioning
Exfoliant, 154

Cucumber De-Puffer Spa Water, 169

Detoxifying Seaweed Body Wrap,
160–61

Fizzy Mojito Foot Spa, 162

Glowing Goddess Face and Body
Mask, 152

Head-to-Toe Pumpkin Mask, 150–51

Jasmine Hair Finishing Oil, 166

Quick Coconut Cantaloupe Cooler,
172

Rosy Green Tea Spa Water, 173

Soothing Scalp and Hair Treatment,
164–65

Strawberry Super C Sipper, 170

Sunrise Spa Water, 167

Vanilla Isle Perfume, 156

Witch hazel, 145, 213

Y

Yerba Flax Face-Food Mask, 42

Yogurt, 213

Yogurt Lavender Comfort Body Mask
and Bath, 179

Z

Zinc oxide, 9, 213

ABOUT THE AUTHOR

JESSICA RESS is chief formulator, founder, CEO, and SpaGoddess at Angel Face Botanicals, an organic skin care company. A certified aromatherapist, she has a natural talent for blending ingredients to create effective therapeutic skin treatments that are a sensory journey for mind, body, and spirit. Jessica's luxurious spa products incorporate aromatherapy and herbalism, are infused with Reiki Healing Energy, and have been her passion for over twenty years. She lives in the beachside town of Santa Cruz, CA, meditates daily, and practices spiritual healing modalities including Crystal and Sound Healing. Jessica and Angel Face Botanicals have been featured in numerous national publications including *Fast Company*, *Cosmopolitan*, *Harper's Bazaar*, and *Huffington Post*. Learn more at *www.angelfacebotanicals.com*.